No Secret

Adventures in Taking God at His Word

By Sharon McGee Ghassami

Unless otherwise noted, all Scripture quotations are from the King James Version of the Bible.

All Scripture quotations marked AMP are taken from The Amplified Bible, New Testament. Copyright © 1958, 1987 by The Lockman Foundation, La Habra, California.

Scripture quotations marked The Message are taken from THE MESSAGE. Copyright © 1993, 1994, 1995, 1996, 2000, 2001, 2002 by Eugene H. Peterson. Used by permission of NavPress Publishing Group.

All Scripture quotations marked NKJV are taken from the New King James Version of the Bible. Copyright © 1979, 1980, 1982, Thomas Nelson, Inc., Publishers.

All Scripture quotations marked NLT are taken from the Holy Bible, New Living Translation, copyright © 1996. Used by permission of Tyndale House Publishers, Inc., Wheaton, Illinois 60189. All rights reserved.

All Scripture quotations marked ESV are taken from The Holy Bible, English Standard Version. Copyright © 2001 by Crossway Bibles, a division of Good News Publishers.

All Scripture quotations marked NIV are taken from The Holy Bible: New International Version® NIV®. Copyright © 1973, 1978, 1984 by International Bible Society. Used by permission of Zondervan Publishing House. All rights reserved.

All Scripture quotations marked RSV are taken from The Revised Standard Version of the Bible. Copyright © 1946, Old Testament Section. Copyright © 1952 by the Division of Christian Education of the Churches of Christ in the United States of America.

All Scripture quotations marked NASB are taken from The New American Standard Bible. Copyright © 1960,1962, 1963, 1968, 1971, 1972, 1973, 1975, 1977, by the Lockman Foundation. La Habra, California.

The Living Bible copyright © 1971 by Tyndale House Foundation. Used by permission of Tyndale House Publishers Inc., Carol Stream, Illinois 60188. All rights reserved. The Living Bible, TLB, and the The Living Bible logo are registered trademarks of Tyndale House Publishers.

No Secret: Adventures in Taking God at His Word
Copyright © 2015 Sharon McGee Ghassami
ISBN: 978-1-944566-07-4

Bush Publishing & Associates books may be ordered at www.BushPublishing.com or www.Amazon.com. For further information, please contact:

Bush Publishing & Associates
www.BushPublishing.com

Because of the dynamic nature of the Internet, any web address or link contained in this book may have changed since publication and may no longer be valid.

Printed in the United States of America. No portion of this book may be used or reproduced by any means: graphic, electronic or mechanical, including photocopying, recording, taping, or by any information storage retrieval system, without the written permission of the publisher, except in the case of brief quotations embodied in critical articles and reviews.

Table of Contents

Foreword 9
Stubborn Faith 12
All the Time 13
He's Got Your Back 15
The Royal Flush 16
First Responder 17
Avoid the Power of Evil; Rely on the Power of God 19
God Never Changes! 22
Hope for All Idiots 23
Still Beholding His Glory 25
The Wisdom of Men vs. the Power of God 26
Captive Thoughts and Healthy Bodies 28
Keep Yourself from Idols 30
Listen to the Comforter and Live! 31
Who Do We Think We Are? 33
Causes and Effects 34
God Won't Put You on Hold 36
Cross My Heart 37
Some Different "Test Results" for Charlie! 39
Whispers? Or Shouts? 41
Pizza Peter and the Power of Persistence 43

Sons of God	44
The Full Monty!	45
Gods Pleasure!	46
Humility with Boots On!	47
The Bridge to Healing	48
Your Own Personal Nest	49
Mark, the Kick B___ Gospel!	50
Me, Too, and I'll Tell!	51
Boo-boos and Ouwies	53
What's the Price?	54
The Workman is Worthy	55
Be Prepared	56
Steadfast and Stand Fast	58
The Belt of Truth	59
The Belt Again	60
Full Armor Against What?	61
The Breastplate of Righteousness	62
Still Polishing...	63
Get Your Shoes On!	64
Extinguishing Flaming Arrows	65
The Helmet	66
Association Caution!	68
Permanent Promises	70
Hungry for Healing	72
Stubborn Determination from II Kings 4	73
Slap Yourself, and Pay Attention!	75
Turn Can't Into Can	76
Quality Control	78
Ticket to Ride	79
Do Some Yelling!	80

It's Who You Know	81
Healing, Conditional Promises	83
Healing: Claim Your Benefits!	**85**
No Lists, No Arguments, Just Thanksgiving and Praise!	87
Healing, in the Flesh	89
Healing, Antiseptic for Filthy Dreamers	90
Are You in the Right Line?	91
Healing, No Evil; No Fear	92
Thank You!	93
Healing—Ask God First	94
Stop Perishing!	95
The Keys to Your Chariot of Fire	96
Healing… On Easy Street	97
Trust…Direction…Promise	98
Check with a Doctor	99
Put Up or Shut Up, According to His Word	101
First Fruits of Faith	102
Christmas Every Day!	104
Batter Up!	106
Pass/Fail and Graduation	107
A Life Sentence	109
Psalm 91: The Insurance/Assurance Policy	110
The Body, A Sacrifice of Worship	112
Health Assessment!	114
Nancy Drew Investigates	116
We're Number One!!!	118
You'd Better Shop Around!	119
Finding your Ebenezer	121
The Secret of the Only Children	123
Bambi…and You	124

Breaking Ignorant	125
Lead Us Not into Temptation But Deliver Us from Evil…	127
How Do You Know if It's Real?	128
On Earth as it Is in Heaven!	129
And I Don't Mean "Maybe!"	131
Denying Jesus	132
The Evidence: YOU!	134
Sherlock…and You!	135
Chastening for the Clueless	136
No Abracadabra	138
No Laughing Matter?	140
Great News! Cool Water!	142
"I Do It!"	144
Narrow the Choices to Two	146
Rescue the Top for Your Toothpaste!	148
Do I Get it?	150
Memory Work	152
Made to Be Whole	154
Thinking about Your Thinking	155
Right Now	157
Healing—A Little Adjustment	159
Healing—Imagination	161
Healing—Who Is Taking the Lead?	163
Healing—Evidence of Things Seen!	164
This Settles It	166
A Thought Correction Away	168
What Will Make Us Whole?	169
Get Your Big "But" Out of the Way and Stop Slowing Down for Green Lights!	170
The Whole Truth and Nothing But the Truth, So Help Me God	172

The Dangers of Exposure	173
The Power of Faith	175
WEAPONS for Health and Healing	177
John 17—Get Real!	179
Healing—Use the Show Towels!	181
Healing—The Great God of Little Things	183
Get Busy—All Shook Up	184
Busted and Disgusted?	185
Pay Attention = Good Cheer!	186
Healing—Spirit Spell Check	188
Precautionary Measures	189
Who Is in Control?	190
Glory! Isn't That Just the Most Amazing Thing?	191
Voice Recognition	192
Listen and Live!	194
You and DIFFERENT	196
Can You Afford That?	198
Bit Him	200
Faith Facing Facts	201
How to Handle the Bully	203
When Will You Have the Time to Get Healed?	205
Beauty for Ashes	207
Celebrating the Color of Your Eyes!	209
Inventory	211
No Abusive Father	214
Facing the "Why?"	216
Answers that Work	218
Heathen or Healed?	220
Home to Healing	222
Temple Maintenance	223

How Is Your Immune System?	225
Who Is Wiping Your Bottom?	227
There's Always a Reason	229
Error Report	231
Sickness? No, Thank You!	233
The Secret Place	235
Being Dead Is No Excuse	236
The Best Route	238
His Gift, Your Choice—Just Do It.	239
Better Than Wishes!	241
Death	242
The Truth That Shames the Devil	245
Making a List and Checking it Twice!	247
Hearing the Voice	249
Healing—Signed, Sealed, Delivered	251
Test Tube Faith	253
The New Normal!	255
Cling to Grace	256
How Do You Act?	258
Fear Not—The Power Is For You!	259
Dictionary Definition	261
For My Healing Believing Friends	263
Citations	265

Foreword

One day I didn't feel well, due to the effects of the flu I seemed to catch every autumn and every spring. Even so, the ironing had to be done, so I was standing with the iron in one hand while the other was flipping channels on a small black and white television trying to find a program to keep me going. I came across a blond woman who was saying she had learned that she did not have to be sick.

This caught my attention! What on earth did she mean by that? I continued to listen as she told her story. She had learned the "secret" to living in health from the Bible. Now, I had read the Bible all my life, and so had my family, but I did not know about this! I discovered she had simply decided that the Bible was true, so she would read it, believe it, and act on what it said.

When the program was over, I found that I was still standing in the same position, with the iron in one hand and the other hand still on the dial! I called my fiancé Moe and told him what I had heard. He laughed and said that the woman's name was Gloria, and her story had led him to check things out for himself, and recommended that I investigate for myself. That was the beginning of a new way of life for me. I learned that the "secret" was really no secret at all. It is clear, simple and available in black and white for the benefit of any seeking reader.

As my knowledge and understanding grew, I met other people who were from different backgrounds and denominations, but had the mongooses' point of view in common. What is that? Kipling tells us their instinct is to run and find out! How exciting it was to share about this wonderful manifestation of the love of God, and to understand more fully just exactly what Jesus did for us on the cross.

Some people never read the bible. Some people read the bible. Some people read the bible and believe it. Some people read the bible, believe it, and live by it because they believe that God means what He says in the Word.

I was in the third group until one experience in my thirties changed everything. Having been treated for headaches and blurred vision since puberty, the condition had begun to intensify until I had to seek more aggressive medical help. I had been to doctors throughout the preceding years, had prayed asking for help, and had experienced temporary relief. This time, the doctor found a dark shadow on an X-ray that lead to consultations with others, and I was told that I had a brain tumor. Asked to return the next day to meet with the surgeons, the prognosis was grim.

On my way home, I passed by the home of friends who were strong Jewish believers so I stopped to ask them to pray with me. To my astonishment, they were not at all distressed! The husband, Mark, asked me what I wanted to pray for. I said I wanted to ask God to be with me and see me through this experience. He asked if I thought God could do that, and I said yes I did. He then asked me if I thought that same God could heal me. Startled, I said of course He could. Then Mark picked up the bible on his coffee table and proved to me that I had a choice. We prayed together, receiving and agreeing with God's will for my perfect healing. The peace that came over me was extraordinary. That night I slept soundly.

The next day another x-ray was taken and all the doctors gathered around it. They were astonished, because there was no shadow, no tumor. They kept looking at the first and then the second x-ray and at me. I was beaming! It was not so much that I was healed, but more that I had discovered what it meant to fully receive the promises of the Word, and the power of the God Who loved me in my own flesh!

From that moment everything changed. Whenever sickness attacked me, I knew I had a choice—from a headache or a sore throat to more serious threats—I could refuse to participate because the source of these attacks was a defeated foe and I knew that in all things, because of my Redeemer, I could be victorious.

Eventually, I began an online conversation about healing, where we could share questions and testimonies. I began posting a "Healing

Team" message almost every day about what we had learned. The team grew rapidly as we shared with interested friends, until finally someone said, "Why don't you put the messages in a book?" So, here it is.

Dedicated with gratitude and love to Gloria Copeland, who opened the door. To Moe Ghassami, who became my husband and living example. To all of the original healing team members: Peggy, Pam, Wallace, Johanna, James, Lulu, Maggie, Odell, Robin, Kelly, Chrissy, Jim, Monica, Annamae, Ruth, Barb, Lisa, Marcello, Joanna, and Cheryl.

My prayer is that you will check it out for yourself. You don't have to be convinced of anything right now, not even of God and His love for you. If you will just check it out, He will reveal Himself to you. That's what He has been longing to do, and that is no secret!

Stubborn Faith

Our healing focus is based solidly on the foundation of faith. We believe that 1) God is GOOD, 2) that God wants us WELL, and that 3) scripture backs this conviction up 100%. Simple, but profound! Taken in faith, the results are victorious beyond all unbelief. We refuse to believe any less than God's best for us: spirit, soul, and body.

Speaking of which, have you ever seen a child, under the demands of the body, throw a fit? Not a pretty sight! How about a child under the demands of the soul (reason/mind/emotions)? Also, not good. Well, it's not any better, and even more dangerous, for adults.

However, the believer who keeps his or her soul and body under the spiritual control of faith walks in what the world calls "miracles" every day of his or her life. I call them miracles too, but I expect them as a normal part of my life! Scripture tells me that the righteousness of God is revealed from faith to faith and the just shall live by faith (Romans 1:17), not the limitations of the body or the realm of reason. We walk by faith, not by sight (II Corinthians 5:7) and we are fully aware of what it is our RIGHT through the blood of Jesus. The stubborn woman of Canaan in Matthew 15:22-28 is our girl! Jesus told her, "O woman, great is thy faith: be it unto thee as thou wilt."

Sign me up for that! Speaking of signs, Jesus told us that through our spreading of the gospel to a needy world, signs and wonders would follow, as a sort of advertisement that what we have is not just wishful thinking!

"Lord, thank you for your love for us. Thank you for revealing your powerful will concerning our walk in the flesh as well as in the soul and spirit. Thank you for forgiving us when we slip, and behave like children who don't know any better. We know better! We know YOU! Help us to be walking advertisements for your victorious love today and always. In Jesus' Name, trusting in Him. Amen!"

All the Time

One of the biggest stumbling blocks that prevent people from receiving healing is also one of the first pieces of information we teach little children.

I remember a Sunday School that I attended had a marvelous way of making scripture impactful. All the classes met in a middle space to pray and praise, and then we divided up into our various classrooms, which branched off from the open space. Every Sunday we learned a scripture and an explanation about what it meant. Then at the end, we'd all come out to the common area and class by class recite our scripture, and the minister would question us about it.

The second scripture the little ones learned was "Jesus went about doing good." They'd recite that, and then they were asked, "Just SOME of the time, or ALL of the time?" and they'd shout back, "ALL THE TIME!" "For SOME people, or for ALL people?" and they'd shout, "For ALL people!" Then, "Are we supposed to be like Jesus?" "YES!!!" "When?" "ALL THE TIME!"

That was the second scripture. The first one they taught to little toddlers, some still in diapers, who were just learning to talk, was "GOD is LOVE." They were asked, "Does He just love some of us?" "NO! ALL of us!" then "Does He love us just some of the time, or ALL of the time?" The whole room would explode, "ALL THE TIME!"

If we understood and believed those two simple scriptures, it would be very hard for our enemy to lay sickness and disease on us. Here are the scriptures (In other words, I AM NOT MAKING THIS UP!):

Acts 10:38 tells "…how God anointed Jesus of Nazareth with the Holy Ghost and with power—who WENT ABOUT DOING GOOD, and healing all that were oppressed of the devil; for God was with Him."

"He that does not love does not know God; for GOD IS LOVE."(John 4:7-9)

People are always telling me, "Well, you have to read scripture in context." I dare you! Go ahead and read it in context and then go LIVE IT IN CONTEXT, the context of your own life. WARNING: these two little scriptures are powerful. If you receive and believe them like those little babies, you won't be able to put up with being sick any more!

He's Got Your Back

I just love to spend time in Matthew Chapter 9. Jesus goes about doing good, ALL the time! His responses to people's needs remind me of a friend of ours named Rocky. Whenever a woman or girl asks him to do something, he always says, "Sure, Shug!" (For you Yankees, that's "Sure, Sugar.") For guys, he says, "OK buddy, I got your back."

Clearly, Jesus was telling the woman with the issue of blood "Sure, Shug," when she was healed through touching His garment. He also gave her an extra gift. He told her that it was her FAITH that made her whole. In other words, her faith would be with her always, even when Jesus was not physically available to her.

It's interesting that He paused for this encounter while on the way to heal someone else, actually to raise the ruler's dead daughter. The father confessed that if Jesus would lay His hand on her, the child would live again. Jesus had his back! He wasn't hurried; He had time for the woman to interrupt Him and get healed. He wasn't all in a dither about the interruption. After all, the child was already dead. However, the father and Jesus both knew, and agreed, that even death could be overcome in this situation, and they were both right. Funny how often we're right when we agree with Jesus!

He goes out of His way to tell us He's got our back, and our kidneys and our hearts and our liver and our head and foot and sore toe! He doesn't pick and choose whom He'll love. Like I learned in Sunday school, it's because God is Love that Jesus went about doing good.

So relax, Shug! Walk in faith! He's got your back!

The Royal Flush

The following is part of an email I received in response to one of the email lessons I taught. My friend, Chrissy, discusses the messages daily with her daughter, Maddie, whom she is home schooling.

"What a wonderful devotion this became for Maddie and me this morning! I woke up and headed down the steps with some heel pain." (Note: Chrissy was delivered from this issue some time ago). "I immediately told that pain, 'NO WAY! Get out!' And it went!"

Maddie then told her mother about a little friend, Shawn, who when scared or sick, immediately told Satan he was flushing him down the toilet. And he flushed him! Everyone needs to "FLUSH" Satan and his sneaky, stupid games! Thank you, Chrissy and Maddie, for taking the time to impact us through that story. The truth is spreading through the generations.

Getting the message to children is so much easier than getting it to hard headed adults. What is it that makes us resist receiving the gifts God has given us so freely? Why do we cling to keeping control over things that God is eager to handle for us in His strength, rather than leaving us helpless to rely on our own?

Do you know what gifts belong to you as a child of God? Go to I Corinthians Chapter 12 to find the 9 Gifts of the Holy Spirit. Paul urges us to "covet earnestly the best gifts." Trust me, your enemy will try to convince you they're not for you. In that case, you may want to join Shawn in some flushing!

Although all the gifts can help us be healed and whole, three in a row, faith, healing, and the working of miracles, are especially powerful for our focus. Do your homework. Be fully persuaded that I am not putting you on!

Also be fully persuaded with childlike faith that God is able to perform ALL that He promises. When we realize the full implication of what it means to be a child of God, sons and daughters of the King, the term "royal flush" takes on a whole new meaning!

First Responder

We are hearing a great many examples of people in peril on the news recently, and the clips usually include the actions of the first responders, the people who immediately go into action when they receive a cry for help.

Who is your first responder? When you are up against it, either suddenly, or in the face of something you've feared would happen for a long time, who ya gonna call? Ghost busters?

Unless that's the HOLY GHOST, you're probably still in big trouble. There is God, holding you in the palm of His Hand, and you call your sister-in-law? Or your goofy cousin, Larry, or that best bud who always gets you into trouble, or Aunt Thelma who is always stressed with drama and lives from one crisis to the next? Of course, we may turn to more sensible choices, but even so, which of them knows more than GOD?

Parents are often horrified to learn that a child has been in trouble or danger, but instead of turning to Dad and Mom they went to another clueless kid. How do you suppose God feels when we, His beloved children, turn to many other sources for help before we finally in desperation turn to Him?

Matthew 6:33 advises us to seek the kingdom of God FIRST, and His righteousness and promises that then "all these things will be given" to us. What are the "things"?? The things we need! When we are sick or sorry, as Granny used to call it, He wants to be our first responder!

Verses 25-34 warn against worry; a sin, which in itself can bring on illness and suffering even when there is no physical basis for it. Verse 32 assures us that our heavenly Father knows our needs, and He is always present and at the ready. No 911 call or sirens, just our Abba/Daddy there to pick us up and make everything all right.

Another benefit is that the insurance won't cost you a dime. It only requires your faith.

"Heavenly Father, Thank you for holding us close in Your protective love, even when we fail to turn to You. Forgive us for forgetting Your promises in moments of fear and panic and pain. Please help us to think of You FIRST every single time, never doubting that You know our needs and are eager to fulfill them out of Your boundless, eternal love. In Jesus' name, amen."

Avoid the Power of Evil; Rely on the Power of God

This title sounds pretty simple and obvious, doesn't it? Taking a closer look at what's floating around our culture can open our eyes to subtle evil we fail to identify accurately, and can affect us and our health without our recognizing what has happened.

There are only two sources of supernatural power in this earth: God and His holy angels, and the devil and his unholy angels. Obviously God is infinitely more powerful and all things will come under the subjection of the Lord Jesus Christ. (Matt. 22:44; I Cor. 15:24-25; Heb. 2:8).

Desperate people try to replace or combine the power of God with demonic "magic arts." These are hideously dangerous and open the door to all kinds of evil, often manifested in illness. They are forbidden to us in order to keep us under the protection of the power of God.

We need not fear these things because Jesus has overcome all of this mess. However, we do need to know what they are and teach our children to avoid them. If you innocently, or even not so innocently, participated in any of these practices, simply go to God and sincerely repent. We need to arm our children against these things, not to frighten them, but to empower them. They need to know that Jesus is Lord!

Here are the evils that are forbidden to us:

1) Occult activities including divination, witchcraft, and astrology Deut. 18:9-13
2) Astrology, seeking information from the stars Isaiah 47:13-14
3) Charms, items worn for their "magical powers"
4) Cursing to do another harm Deut. 28:15-68; Matt. 21:118-21; I Sam. 17:43; I Kings 19:2
5) Divination, the practice of foreseeing or foretelling future events

6) Consulting "familiar spirits", dead people evoked by a medium for consultation or a demon invoked (demons are not born and do not die Luke 20:36, Deut. 18:20-22; 29
7) Consulting a fortuneteller who claims to know the future via tea leaves or reading palms, etc.
8) Speaking or picturing a hex (or jinx) over someone, casting an evil spell, curse, or bad luck on another person; to practice witchcraft or sorcery
9) Consulting or acting as a "medium", someone who is "in-between" and communicates with the dead or supernatural agents.
10) Necromancy, black art which contacts the dead for consultation or divination I Samuel 28:7-25
11) Clairvoyants or psychics I Samuel 9:9
12) Sorcery, using ungodly supernatural powers Exodus 7:11; Acts 8:9-13 and 16.
13) Spell, word or formula believed to have magical powers
14) Spiritists, supposed to be able to communicate with the dead
15) Witchcraft, often called "The Craft"; or "Wicca," the current spin on this, packaged as a pagan nature religion from pre-Christian Western Europe. It is now experiencing a 20th century revival. (Swell, as if we didn't have enough to get us in trouble!)

You have no doubt encountered some of this yourself. If you haven't, just turn on the TV for a few minutes! To keep ourselves out of darkness and walking in the light of God's power and mercy, we need to see all of these things for what they are, and cast them out of our lives.

The good news is the battle has already been won! Hooray! How do we know?

1) Jesus has defeated the devil! (I John 3:8; Acts 10:38; Heb. 2:14-15; John 1:3; John 12:27; Col. 2:10 and 2:15; Mark 1:21-27; 3:11; 5:7; Luke 4:34; Mark 4:39-41)
2) Because we acknowledge Jesus as Lord, we share His victory and find our safety in His righteousness through faith and trust in Him alone. (Eph. 2:1-2;8-10; I John 2:22-23; II Cor. 5:17; Col. 1:13-14, Eph. 5:8; I Cor. 6:9-11).
3) We are now people of God, who are equipped to resist the devil! Look these up and prove it to yourself: James 4:7-8; Eph. 6: 12-13;

I John 4:4; Mark 1:27; Rom. 8:31-39; III John 11; Acts 19:19 (where they burned those magic books) and Romans 12:21.

More good news: we do not need to fear any of these evils! Just avoid them and refuse to participate in them. The Devil and his demonic forces fear God. They know they are under God's wrath. They know they are a defeated, pitiful foe.

I personally am convinced that sickness and disease are evil things and not the will of God. I walked in ignorance about these things quite innocently for a long time, BUT NOT ANY MORE! I am equipped with the truth, Praise God! How about you?

God Never Changes!

One of the most wonderful things about God is that He never changes. His love and care and mercy are always the same, at all times, for all people who will receive them. What a sense of security we can have in Him; how wholeheartedly we can trust Him! All those healing promises, all the stories of how He healed person after person, all of that has not changed. All of that is for you and me right now. "We thank you and praise you for that Lord! Please help us to walk in that certainty."

You probably know the song...but today might be a good time to hum it or even sing it:

Oh how sweet to trust in Jesus,
Just to take Him at His word,
Just to rest upon the promise;
Just to know "Thus saith the Lord."

Jesus, Jesus, how I trust you,
How I've proved you o'er and o'er!
Jesus, Jesus, precious Jesus
Oh for faith to trust you more.[1]

How wonderful if when sickness or disease or injury tries to attack, that melody would be the first thing that comes to mind! How about if we remembered first and last, "I am the Lord, I change not." (Malachi 3:6)

Hope for All Idiots

I guess it should be comforting to us that people have behaved like idiots even in the presence of God's mercy throughout the ages. There it is, that eternal mercy that wants to bless us, that longs to give us every good and perfect gift! We want to do that for our children and other loved ones, but we commit blasphemy against God when accusing Him of loving us less than we love our own. We accuse Him of wanting us to suffer pain and sickness and poverty. Like I said, THAT is blasphemy!

Need an example? Take a look at Lamentations Chapter 3. This is not a jolly rancher here. Have you ever known someone who just INSISTED on being miserable? The whining and groaning and "poor me" syndrome is so pleasurable in some twisted way that they can't receive any relief. People cling to their misery. They remain drama kings and queens to the end!

When you think about this, don't you just see the little kid throwing a fit? NOTHING you suggest will comfort or calm him down! This one, however, does admit the mercy of God. As he is railing away, we see the undeniable glimpses of light:

"It is because of the Lord's mercies we are not consumed. His compassions fail not. They are new every morning. Great is thy faithfulness! The Lord is my portion, says my soul; therefore I will hope in Him. The Lord is good to those who wait on Him, to the soul that seeks Him" (verses 22-25).

Does it seem cruel to compare the determination of a child throwing a tantrum to the believer clinging to illness and other miseries? Does that seem to be blaming the victim? Honestly, I used to think that, and I was indignant that anyone would suggest such a thing.

However, I was walking in ignorance, an idiot in the face of the truth of God's wonderful will for me, and for all of us. Once I could truly embrace the fact that the most powerful God of the universe loved me and wants nothing but the divine best for me, I repented in ashes and dust, as Job puts it. Once I had identified my enemy accurately and realized that it is NOT GOD, I got the picture and determined I would no longer blaspheme God!

Praise God for His mercies that are new every morning, and His infinite patience that faithfully embraces us until we are ready to receive His victorious love. When we catch ourselves being attacked by the promised tribulation from many fronts, it's time to wake up and remember our rights and run to the mercy that is new for us. They are new every morning.

Still Beholding His Glory

John 1:14 "And the Word was made flesh and dwelt among us, and we beheld His glory..."

Did you ever receive one of those goofy emails that promised all kinds of good things if and only if you passed it on to 10 people? Or warned of terrible things happening to you if you refused? Or both? Did you ever read a "tip" of some little thing you could do that would cure, reduce, solve something and buy into it? Did you ever really believe something was true just because you read it online or heard it repeated by several people?

Sadly, people do this, while they ignore the one thing that will deliver on promises and truly avoid disasters: the Word of God!

For me, the dealmaker is John 1:14. When Jesus took on a physical body and showed us IN THE FLESH what we could do IN THE FLESH, people beheld His Glory.

At our church, we have been praying for two people having inoperable brain tumors. In both cases the family has "known" (rather, been told!) that these tumors can, on rare occasions, be in remission but will never shrink. Guess what? Without knowing it in advance, BOTH of these families arrived at Sunday worship to report that BOTH tumors are shrinking! The doctors are stunned and are scrambling to record the test results, as this is unprecedented! It's hard to tell who's more thrilled: the patients, the families, or the praying believers at church. Rejoice with us; what a mighty God we serve!

You see, we beheld His Glory today. We, too, saw as the Word made someone's flesh healthy, victorious, and tumor-defeating.

I'll take a pass on the goofy emails and the Internet tips. I'm banking on the source that keeps promises: Jesus, the same yesterday, today and forever. How about you?

The Wisdom of Men vs. the Power of God

"That your faith might not rest in the wisdom of men, but in the power of God." I Corinthians 2:5

"Have you listened in on the counsel of God? And do you limit wisdom to yourself?" Job 15:8

One morning, I received an email from someone I love who is not a believer. Her lifestyle choices, including those concerning health and wellness, are made according to a mixture of worldly "wisdom," science (when it agrees with her views), and her own ideas. For thirty years she has maintained this perspective and for thirty years she has experienced health issues one after another. Yet she maintains, "I have a healthy life," and reports that recent medical tests confirm that. "At least according to the way I choose to interpret those tests," she said.

The fact that we are all in life where we are to a large extent because of the choices we have made is a tough reality, but looking at results is a great diagnostic tool. We need to ask, "Is this working or is this NOT working?"

We've all heard the saying, "If it ain't broke, don't fix it" and "Insanity is continuing to do the same thing over and over and expecting different results." These are, of course, also examples of worldly wisdom, perhaps in the category of "horse sense" or "mother wit."

The point? We need to take a hard look at the results of our choices and check the results. If they are not what we want or need, it would be an excellent idea to see if they line up with what GOD says.

As believers, we are privy to divine information that is readily available to us at all times to guide our steps in this temporary, material world. How do we "choose to interpret the tests?" The passage from Job warns of the foolishness of interpreting through our own wisdom when the counsel of God is an alternative choice! Does this mean we have to reject the wisdom of men? Of course not, AS LONG AS IT LINES UP WITH THE WISDOM OF GOD.

Of course, the power of God and His wisdom is beyond anything we can grasp fully, but we can, nevertheless, access it freely because He loves us! His strength is available to us in our weakness, but **we must choose** to seek and receive it. What are YOUR test results? If they are not what you want, check your sources and your resources! Go to God in scripture and in prayer. Know what you'll find out? It's in that simple Sunday School song:

> "Jesus loves me, this I know
> For the Bible tells me so,
> Little ones to Him belong;
> They are weak, but He is strong." [2]

Cling to that, and your whole being, spirit, soul, and body, will pass the test every time.

Captive Thoughts and Healthy Bodies

"Though we walk in the flesh we do not war after the flesh, for the weapons of our warfare are not carnal (physical) but mighty through God to the pulling down of strongholds; casting down imaginations and every thing that exalts itself against the knowledge of God, and bringing into captivity every thought to the obedience of Christ." (II Corinthians 10:3-5).

There is a LOT in this scripture that reveals important truth concerning health and healing.

First of all, even though we are *in* bodies, the bodies are not really the issue. Did you ever hear someone say that sin doesn't begin with an action, it begins with a thought? We can probably all agree with that! But what about disease, illness, accidents, allergies, and so on? Here we learn that we must cast down "imaginations" that can become strongholds in our minds.

An interesting experiment tested this. I learned about it in a psychology class in college where perfectly healthy people were told by several others, "You look like you don't feel well today." "Are you coming down with something?" "You look flushed, do you have a fever?" By the end of the day, they were all sick. The thought was planted, their imaginations took over and then their bodies followed right along.

Did you ever register with a new doctor and have to fill out that form about "family history?" You are asked to list all the diseases and conditions of everyone in your family SO THAT THE DOCTOR CAN BE AWARE OF THEM WHEN TREATING YOU. He is ANTICIPATING WHAT MIGHT BE IN STORE FOR YOU!

I'll never forget the glorious day Moe and I realized we didn't have to have ANY of the items on that list! No, they just didn't line up with the Word of God and His will for our health. We decided we would agree with Him, not our family history. It was one of the best decisions we ever made! We became part of the Body of Christ and we have **none of those diseases!** (Exodus 15:26) Since that day, NONE of those diseases!!! Halleluiah! What's my track record? Thirty plus years and going strong!

Notice the use of the word "Christ" in the scripture from II Corinthians. This term refers to Jesus and His anointing. That anointing power is available to us through Him. We can walk in it, shelter in it, and be safe in it. Best of all, in the strength of it, we can cast down those strongholds that have taken hold in our minds, especially FEAR (false evidence appearing real) and with the help of Jesus bring our thoughts into the obedience of agreeing with Him.

God has provided a way for us to live in the flesh in a fallen world and still be healthy. That way includes rejecting every thought and imagination that stands in contradiction to God's healing, victorious love for you, and imagining yourself strong and whole in every way, every minute, all the time. Just imagine!

Keep Yourself from Idols

We know that the son of God is come, and has given us understanding so that we can know what is true, and we are in Him who is true in His son Jesus Christ. This is the true God, and eternal life. Little children, keep yourselves from idols. Amen" (I John 5:20-21).

Verse 21 had always puzzled me. Coming as it does at the end of a remarkable chapter in a remarkable book of scripture, it seemed like an oddly abrupt little statement, and I certainly never saw its significance in terms of healing or health. Today it hit me! How? THE RAVENS WON!

Let me explain. Before the big game here in Maryland, it was all about the Ravens. The chatter, the speculation, even the bets! People planned PARTIES to get together to watch the game! Then there were victory parties! People WORE PURPLE before, during, and after the game and the win.

In the middle of this, as I shared in a previous message, two people received the victory of shrinking tumors. The reaction of "the crowd?" Some polite clapping (Brief! Controlled! Restrained!) and maybe a hug or two. Now I ask you, what was the greater victory? God's miracles are happening all around us, but they get very little press. Do we anticipate them? Expect them? Talk to everyone about them? Celebrate them when they happen? Or are we so busy and focused on sporting events or American Idol (oops!) that we fail to seek, honor, and celebrate the TRUTH?

In a peculiar irony, on the day of the game, the clergy were also wearing purple stoles in church because of the beginning of the season of Lent, a season of reflection and repentance.

Verse 20 reminds us of why Jesus came, and how He brought understanding to us so that we could know what is true.

May I suggest that we repent of ignoring that truth, caught up in the distractions of this world to the degree that we have no time to seek and grasp and celebrate the priceless miracles He offers through His love? Do we really want to walk in health? In victory? Then TRUTH is going to have to be more important and more exciting than a Ravens' game. Little children, keep yourselves from idols. Now that's a kickoff!

Listen to the Comforter and Live!

"I call heaven and earth to record this day against you, that I have set before you life and death, blessing and cursing: therefore choose life, that both thou and thy seed may live" (Deuteronomy 30:19)

"And if it seem evil unto you to serve the Lord, choose you this day whom ye will serve; whether the gods which your fathers served that were on the other side of the flood, or the gods of the Amorites, in whose land ye dwell: but as for me and my house, we will serve the Lord." (Joshua 24:14)

"Nevertheless I tell you the truth; It is expedient for you that I go away: for if I go not away, the Comforter will not come unto you; but if I depart, I will send Him unto you." (John 16:7).

"But the Comforter, which is the Holy Ghost, whom the Father will send in my name, He shall teach you all things, and bring all things to your remembrance, whatsoever I have said unto you" (John 14:26)

So much of the power of what we have been studying about healing depends upon the source we each select as the foundation for our belief. I know that sometimes some of you may read something I've stated in a message, and ask, "Sharon! ARE YOU TELLING ME that...?"

No, I am not. What I am telling you is what the Word is telling ME! God is not confused or varying. What the Word tells one of us, it tells all of us. Do people interpret it differently? Sure they do! We humans are good at "picking and choosing." We are always wanting things to agree with our own ideas. How can we get around that and get at the real truth?

Other people are thinking, "Well sure, Jesus healed when He was on the earth, but now He is gone, so we can't expect to be healed that way now." That does not line up with what scripture says! No matter how many people have thought this and said it, it does not agree with scripture.

Jesus told His flock that when He left He would send the Holy Spirit. He said that all He had spoken to them came from His FATHER who dwelt in Him, and that when He left earth those who believe on Him will do the same works that He did and EVEN GREATER WORKS. He says (John 14:13-18) that the Holy Spirit will dwell in us forever. Verses 13-14 even say that anything we ask in His Name He will do, so that the Father may be glorified.

Check it out for yourselves. I am not making it up. Sometimes people say to me, "Well, I don't see it that way..." Do you know, if we read the same scripture and ask the Holy Spirit to reveal the truth to us He will tell us both the same thing?

The sticking point is that WE have the choice. What are we going to believe? That boils down to WHO we are going to believe. Have you figured out that not all "opinions" have the same value? The day I took God at His WORD, I asked the Holy Spirit to teach me as I read the scripture. Immediately, everything changed.

So I say to you, just like Joshua said, "Choose today." Believe Him, and you won't have to wonder any more.

Who Do We Think We Are?

When we boldly insist on receiving the promises of God, people sometimes get really irritated. They say, "Just who do you think you are?" Do we think for some reason we have a RIGHT to victory? Health? Joy? YEP! We do! Drives the world, and even some believers, nuts.

Why? Because we know who we are! We know from Genesis who God created us to be. He created us people in His own image, created to live a life of total blessing in the garden, fellowshipping with Him. We also know how we lost it, don't we? But here's the kicker, we should ALSO KNOW HOW WE GOT IT BACK.

If we ignore the victory Jesus won for us on the cross, He might as well have opted out. If we ignore the indwelling of the Holy Spirit, whom He sent to minister to us after He left the earth, the Holy Spirit might as well not have come. Christmas is just all about snowmen, Christmas trees, and shopping, as the heathens would have us believe, and Pentecost just a day to wear red. Deal with it! What is the truth? Face it and move forward!

Who are we? Don't ask your best bud or your worst enemy or your brother-in-law, ask God. We are:

1) "Heirs of God and joint heirs with Christ" (Romans 8:17)
2) "More than conquerors through Him that loved us" (Rom. 8:37)
3) Those whose physical bodies can be healed: "If the Spirit that raised up Jesus from the dead dwells in you, then He that raised up Christ from the dead will also quicken your mortal body by His Spirit that dwells in you! (Rom 8:11)"

Let me ask you something: Is there ANYTHING you were planning to do today that is more important than walking in your inheritance as a healed conqueror?

I didn't think so. Alleluia!

Causes and Effects

Most people, I expect, first think of sickness and disease as physical pain or discomfort or injury. Some of these we experience as children and have obvious causes: you fall down, and scrape your knee; you catch a cold/measles/flu from someone who is coughing and hacking, etc. The cause and effect are fairly clear. We don't ask, "But WHY did I fall down, WHY was Billy coughing, WHY did I catch it and my sister didn't?" Not yet.

Then we grow older and observe or experience personally diseases with origins not so easily discernable, and we begin to ask, "Why her? Why me?"

In both cases, we assume there IS A CAUSE, and this is the spark that fires medical research and science. Maybe, we reason, if we can determine the cause, then we can fix it.

Then we realize that there are also diseases of the mind, or at least the brain. The brain is material. It can be examined and probed and explored. The mind is something else. Many documented cases show that people who have experienced severe brain trauma and/or go into comas and then recover share with us that they were conscious the whole time. The brain registered "off" but the mind was still working! This should give us pause for serious thinking.

Many people fear mental illness even more than physical illness. We cry out with King Lear: "O, let me not be mad, not mad, sweet heaven, Keep me in temper: I would not be mad." (King Lear, Scene V). We watch loved ones age, and wish for them an alert mind till the end, feeling that in this way they are still "with us."

Cause and effect are serious considerations. Science declares "Matter is neither created nor destroyed," and if we listen carefully there is an eternal answering whisper "...by man." "Nothing comes from nothing" resonates with us.

This sense, so inherent in mankind and so universal, has great implications for us as believers, and scripture backs it. There is a cause for everything. Causes have effects. That is why the choices made, as we walk through this life with free will, are so important. They are important because every choice we make becomes a cause that will have an effect. We must learn to be wise enough to choose CONSEQUENCES instead of just choosing actions!

If you've stayed with me this far, you "no doubt" have the sense that this is a thundering great dilemma for us. How do we do it? We must remember…"And the WORD became flesh, and dwelt among us**…**"(John 1:14) and also**,** "God so loved the world that He gave His only begotten son…"(John 3:16). If we can remember and understand the great implication of that glorious reality with "no doubt" we can question fearlessly about the causes of sickness, whether mental or physical. The God who took on flesh to show us how, the God who created us and gave His son, the God who seeks to enter into us, will show us the answers.

One tip: We need to focus less on the causes of our enemy, our ONLY enemy, and more on the God who can make us glorious, spirit, soul and body, in this world and forever.

God Won't Put You on Hold

Moe came home from errands one day and walked in to a house smelling delicious from pot roast and vegetables cooking on the stove. He reacted immediately! He didn't talk about how good it smelled or how hungry he was, he just got the plates and forks out and dove right in! After all, wasn't that why I cooked it in the first place? Why wait?

For the most part, that is the way God operates with His blessings for us. We don't have to long for them from afar! We need to check them out. With very few exceptions, in the Bible people got action immediately. Search the scriptures for yourself. You don't find Jesus putting people on hold! They ask for healing, He provides it, and they receive it and go on their way rejoicing.

On occasion, someone is asked to do something in the process. For example, Namaan had to dip in the muddy Jordan River, and one blind man needed two applications of mud. However, usually the healing was immediate. We hear people say, "Well, sometimes it happens that way, but sometimes God chooses to do it gradually over time." I'm not sure where that came from, but I can find no examples in scripture. I've seen people receive their healing like that myself. I'm sure there are reasons for that, but are they God's reasons or our own?

Many prayers sincerely offered are answered in "God's time," meaning the prime time for the request to be granted because God can see how the consequences will fit into His eternal plan, and we can't. Because I see the immediate relief examples in the cases of Jesus healing, and I want to be like Jesus, I am voting for immediate. But that's just me!

One thing I know for sure, God NEVER puts us on hold. His love has no time limits. It is the immediate relief you can always expect, every single time. Receive it, and go on your way rejoicing!

Cross My Heart

When you were a kid, did you and your friends test your truthfulness by reciting, "Cross my heart and hope to die. Stick a needle in my eye?" That was the ultimate, serious statement that at least THIS time the person reciting it was speaking the truth!

It was necessary, because for much of the time lies were a part of the conversation. You learned fairly quickly who was a truthful friend and who was not, but under extreme conditions, the convicted little liars repeated the mantra to stress that THIS TIME they really were telling the truth!

Who do we believe? This is an interesting and critical question for us as adults, because lying and false information, whether mistaken or intentional, is rampant. Turn on the TV and watch prominent people lie with total conviction. When the truth is revealed, it seems to be received with a shrug as though honesty was not really expected.

I was a very fortunate child in that my parents always told me the truth. They were the source I could always trust 100% of the time. They, in turn, trusted the Word of God, grounded in the fact that it never failed them. Trusting in the Word became a part of me. No friends, teachers, athletes or rock stars were ever as consistently truthful as my parents!

Mark Chapter 6 tells an interesting story of Jesus the Healer going to visit His hometown, clearly hoping to bless the people there as He has blessed so many others with His healing ministry. But no! The folks there were having no part of it. They asked, "'Is this not the carpenter, the Son of Mary, and brother of James, Joses, Judas, and Simon? And are not His sisters here with us?' So they were offended at Him." (Mark 6:3) Jesus explains that one may be honored for His work elsewhere, but not in His own house, and He grieves that He is only able to heal a few.

Who can you trust most? Who is the proven resource you can trust all the time? For some, it may be a family member, teacher, clergyman or friend. For others these sources are not consistently reliable.

It is absolutely critical to discover the trustworthy, consistently truthful resource you can count on every single time. Your life will depend upon it.

For me, that is Jesus, every single time. If you are searching, I highly recommend you check Him out. You will never be disappointed. Cross my heart!

Some Different "Test Results" for Charlie!

When praying healing for someone who believes God can heal him, I always want to be sure I am praying "correctly" based on what scripture really says. To help keep me on track, I put together a list of scripture to create a prayer. You will find it here with the name of Charlie, but you can insert the name of any person for whom you pray.

1) Charlie's faith is the substance of things hoped for; the evidence of things not seen. (Heb. 11:1)
2) Jesus Himself took Charlie's infirmities and bore his sickness. (Matt.8:17)
3) Whatsoever things Charlie asks, when he prays, believing that he receives them, he shall have them (Mark 11:24).
4) Jesus gave His apostles power and delegated authority over all devils, and to cure diseases, including Charlie's! (Luke 9:1-2) They took that authority and "healed everywhere" (Luke 9:6).
5) Jesus said, "These signs shall follow them that believe, in My Name they shall lay hands on the sick, and they shall recover" (Mark 16:15-18).
6) Jesus said, "Behold, I give you power to tread on serpents and scorpions, and over ALL THE POWER OF THE ENEMY: and NOTHING shall by any means hurt you" (Luke 10:19).
7) Greater is He that is in Charlie, than He who is in the world (John 4:4).
8) If Charlie asks any thing in Your Name, You will do it. (John 14:13-14).
9) With His stripes Charlie is healed. With His stripes Charlie was healed. (Is. 53:5; I Peter 2:24).
10) Is Charlie sick? Call for the elders of the church and let them pray for him, anointing him with oil in the name of the Lord: and

the prayer of faith shall save him, and the Lord will raise him up (James 5:14-15).
11) Jesus bore Charlie's sicknesses for him! (Matt. 8:17).
12) Charlie shall come to his grave in a full age like a shock of corn comes in its season (Job 5:26) after living a fruitful life (Ps. 92:14) fulfilling the number of his days (Ex.23:26) until he shall be forever with the Lord (I Thess. 4:17).
13) Because Charlie has set his love upon You, therefore You will deliver him: You will set him on high, because he has known Your Name. He shall call upon You, and you will answer him: You will be with him in trouble; You will deliver him, and honor him. With long life will You satisfy him, and show him my salvation (Ps. 91:14-16).
14) "My covenant with Charlie I will not break, nor alter the thing that has gone out of my lips." (Ps. 89:34)
15) Jesus Christ the same yesterday, and today, and forever! (Heb.3:8)

By the way, Charlie is healed!

Whispers? Or Shouts?

Were you ever praying for healing, for yourself or someone else, and the little whispers of doubt began to distract you? "Does God's will for healing really apply in this case? Am I doing the right thing? What if I do it wrong and it doesn't work?" Those whispers can steal your concentration, your power, and the victory if you're not careful.

To arm you against this nonsense, below are some supporting scriptures to speak when in prayer for healing. These are not whispers, cowardly little whispers, my friend. No, these are SHOUTS!! These are shouts down through the ages and into eternity, shouts of praise! Grab hold of them and you'll automatically drown out the whispers. They won't stand a chance!

Scriptures to support prayers for healing and health:

"Bless the Lord, O my soul, and forget not all His benefits: who forgives all your iniquities; who heals all your diseases; who redeems your life from destruction; who crowns you with loving kindness and tender mercies; who satisfies your mouth with good things; so that your youth is renewed like the eagle's." (Ps. 103:1-5)

"Heal me, O Lord, and I shall be healed; save me, and I shall be saved: for thou art my praise." (Jer. 17:14)

"For I will restore health to you, and I will heal you of your wounds, says the Lord" (Jer. 30:17).

"Jesus Christ, the same yesterday, and today, and forever" (Hebrews 13:8).

"Do not be afraid, for I am with you: don't be dismayed; for I am your God: I will strengthen you; yes, I will help you, yes I will uphold you with the right hand of my righteousness" (Isaiah 41:10).

"He was wounded for our transgressions, He was bruised for our iniquities; the chastisement of our peace was upon Him; and with His stripes we are healed" (Is. 53:5).

"And behold, there came a leper and worshipped Him saying, Lord if you will, you can make me clean. And Jesus put forth His hand, and touched him, saying I will, be clean. And immediately his leprosy was cleansed" (Matt.8:16-17).

"And all things whatsoever you ask in prayer, believing, you shall receive" (Matt. 21:22).

"And these signs shall follow those who believe: In my name they shall cast out devils; they shall speak with new tongues; they shall take up serpents; and if they drink any deadly thing, it shall not hurt them; they shall lay hands on the sick and they shall recover" (Mark 16:16-18).

"And the whole multitude sought to touch Him: for there went virtue out of Him, and healed them all" (Luke 6:19).

"There came also a multitude out of the cities around Jerusalem, bringing sick folks, and those who were vexed with unclean spirits: and they were healed every one" (Acts 5:16).

"But if the Spirit of Him that raised up Jesus from the dead dwell in you, He that raised up Christ from the dead shall also quicken your mortal bodies by His Spirit that dwells in you"(Romans 8:11).

"Is any sick among you? Let him call for the elders of the church: and let them pray over him, anointing him with oil in the name of the Lord: And the prayer of faith shall save the sick, and the Lord shall raise him up; and if he has committed sins they shall be forgiven him. Confess your faults to one another, and pray for one another, that you may be healed. The effective fervent prayer of a righteous man avails much" (James 5:14-16).

"Beloved, I wish above all things that you may prosper and be in good health, even as your soul prospers" (3 John: 2).

"Jesus Christ, the same yesterday, and today, and forever"
(Hebrews 13:8).

Pizza Peter and the Power of Persistence

While visiting Peter's family one weekend, his mom started preparing a chicken dinner. Peter remarked that he'd really like to have pizza. She explained that it was going to be chicken this time. He didn't argue, but he kept quietly talking to himself about how good pizza is. He asked me my favorite kind, and asked his mother hers. Pretty soon we could almost smell that pizza! He went on and on and on in that youthful mode. Guess what we had for dinner?

A friend got a revelation about persistence one day when she realized Jesus is never fickle. He doesn't change His mind! She decided to plug herself into Him, regardless of what she saw, heard, or felt. Her husband joined her, and they found out that pure persistence in faith rings the bell every time.

Then they taught their family. Do you know that sickness and disease don't have a chance with these people! I could tell you story after story! Stuff comes against one of them from time to time—scripture warns, "...in this world you will have tribulation..."—but they just won't put up with it. Why? Because the same scripture also says, "...but be of good cheer! I have overcome the world!"

Want to have those same results? Then duplicate my friend's persistence, and Peter's! Just look Satan in the eye and laugh and shout, "Pizza, pizza, pizza!!!" He'll get the message.

Sons of God

This last week we were out of state, meeting with people we have not seen in a while. Some we had prayed over for healing in the past. They reported that not only did they receive their healing then, but that the issue had never returned! Of course, that's exactly what we expect. When we pray to cast out sickness, we also pray that it will never return.

John's gospel tells us, "...to as many as received Him, to them He gave the power to become the sons of God, even to them that believe on His Name..." That would be us, as well as those who saw Him in the flesh. When we receive, we can receive it all! It is POWER we receive.

Don't be afraid of the power of God. Don't be afraid to welcome it into yourself personally. It will trump the power of the enemy, sickness, disease, and any other evil. When you walk in that power, the enemy's power will be revealed as the puny, defeated nonsense it truly is, and you will walk in victory. Guaranteed!

The Full Monty!

Old Testament people knew God as the creator YHWH, as do our Jewish friends. New Testament people met Jesus, and some recognized Him as God, as do our Christian friends. Then the Holy Spirit came to us. What happened? What happens now? Some receive Him, but some have Him on hold.

The power of the Trinity is so glorious. It's hard to believe that anyone would not want to know and see God in His completeness. We show small children ice, water, and steam. They can see that all three are H2O in different forms. Once they understand that example then they can grasp how the Trinity works. Can you imagine enjoying the benefits of water and ice but refusing the steam? Think of hot baths, clean laundry, hot chocolate, think of little Robbie Fulton and his mama's steam kettle!

The Holy Spirit dwelling in you brings healing home, right here, right now, right where we live. He brings healing and counsel and teaching and comfort. They are all available 24/7/365. Why on earth would we back away from that? "Welcome, Holy Spirit! We receive you with gladness and joy! Please enter our hearts and dwell forever! With you, nothing will be impossible for us ever again. Alleluia!"

Gods Pleasure!

When I was little, Mom overheard me one day saying to my dolls, "Your mommy loves you! That's what mommies do, you know, they love their babies!" I've said that to dolls, cats, dogs, and children! That is what mothers and fathers do. They love their children and want only the best for them.

So it is with our Heavenly Father. How it must grieve Him when He is accused of wanting His children to experience pain and sorrow and suffering. How it must hurt when He is accused of being less loving than earthy fathers strive to be with their own children. What a hideous thing to believe about our kind and loving Father!

Jesus calls Him "Abba, Father" meaning "Daddy," that little word of trust and affection that means so much. Paul reminds the Philippians (2:13) that "...it is God who works in you both to will and to do His pleasure." Think about that. His PLEASURE. Is trouble, sorrow, suffering, sickness, poverty and disease the PLEASURE of a loving father? God forbid! His pleasure is all that is good, and perfect, and wonderful for us.

How do we receive these gifts? The scripture says they are works done "in you." It is through us that the indwelling Holy Spirit offers the infinite gifts of His love and tenderness. Our healing and well-being in every aspect is the divine pleasure of our Abba. Let's remember that with joy and power today and always, in Jesus' Name, Amen.

Humility with Boots On!

One morning I received a meditation on the subject of humility, and experienced one of those light bulb moments. Humility does not mean that you have to be a Sweet Sue or a Wimpy Warren! It simply means submission to God. Surely submission to God is one of the most powerful, practical, and intelligent things we can do. Let's have a rousing cheer for humility!

I can wrap myself around this deal, instead of shrinking gently into a corner and being a doormat. I can stand up and be counted as one of the most powerful creatures in the universe because I am in submission to Him. Look out sickness, disease, doubt, fear, want, trouble, and all those curses, I am shaking the humility club in your ugly face, so get running!

Wow! Doesn't that feel great? Receive it, and get with God's REAL vision of the strength He gives you for His purpose in your life. Who knew? It wasn't that you weren't capable after all! Submit and get your club and start swinging!

The Bridge to Healing

Have you ever known anyone who suffered from an illness for years? Who went to many doctors and suffered under treatment? Who spent all they had seeking relief? Have you wondered if maybe there are cases that are hopeless for healing, for reasons we just don't understand?

Really? Does that really sound like God? Go to Mark 5:25-34 to get your groove back.

Jesus has just performed a miracle, and a crowd of people is "thronging" around Him pushing Him from every direction as He moves toward His next destination. Think of the pushing and shoving we sometimes endure to get into a hit show or concert, to get into the after-Christmas sales, to get into the game of the century, we've all been in a throng!

No one was getting healed until suddenly Jesus felt healing virtue move in Him and pass into the body of a woman who had suffered for years as described previously. Jesus asked who touched Him, and His disciples thought he'd lost it, since the whole crowd was touching Him! (I have to say that reading about some of the goofy things the disciples said and did gives me hope for the rest of us.)

Jesus explains that it was HER FAITH that activated His power for her healing. She had tried many other sources in the HOPE that she might find relief, but she KNEW with faith that if she could just touch His garment she would be healed, and so she was.

Her illness was real. The healing power of Jesus was real. Once the bridge of her faith was crossed, she was healed. Jesus told her to go in peace and be whole.

So, what do we do with this? Jesus Christ is the same, yesterday, today, and forever. It's your call!

Your Own Personal Nest

Birds are on my mind these days as we watch them building nests in the most unusual places. One couple has built a nest inside the plastic cover of our grill on the deck (hold the steaks for a few weeks). They carry huge chunks of moss and leaves many times their size and weight. We are amazed at what they accomplish! How is it possible for these tiny creatures?

It's possible because their faith is automatic! Scripture reminds us to consider the birds of the air, and how God has provided for them beyond the provision of the palaces of Solomon. Matthew 6:26 asks us to realize that God provides absolutely everything for them, and asks us why in the world He would not do the same for us. "Are you not of more value than they?"

God gave them, and us, our bodies for this earthly life. He also gives us safety and provision and health. The difference is that we are not on automatic. We have free will, and must choose: will we seek Him, and trust His love for us? Where have you built your nest?

We have built ours in the palm of His hand. We live near His heart, feeling the beat of His great love for us. If He provides so bountifully for all living things, we can trust Him to provide for us. Those little birds don't worry about whether than can carry those loads! They don't stress over how to construct the nest! For them, it's automatic.

So after you struggle to assess health measures and medical plans and insurance and health club membership and prescription co-pays and all that assails you as you attempt to do it on your own...remember the birds! Your own personal nest is waiting for you right in the palm of God's hand.

(Psalm 50:11, Psalm 104:27-28, Matt.10:29, Luke 12:18, Luke 12:24)

Mark, the Kick B___ Gospel!

In the Gospel of Mark scripture clarifies two important things: 1) Satan is the author of sickness/disease/affliction, and 2) the time for the fulfillment of the Kingdom of God had come with Jesus, and we are to repent and believe (Mark 1:15).

Jesus also clearly teaches that Satan will bind us if he can and then destroy us. One of the ways he tries is through sickness, but Jesus can overcome any evil Satan chooses to inflict on us.

The specific conditions are clearly listed: fevers, unclean spirits, diseases, plagues, leprosy, palsy, withered hands, etc. One by one He casts them out. Mark 3:22-27 explains that Satan will use these things to BIND us so that he can SPOIL our house.

Clearly and accurately identifying the source of "tribulations" that come against us, and their purpose, is huge in helping us resist them, fight them, and, through the shed blood of Jesus, overcome them.

We can refuse to be bound! Not through our own grit and determination, not through the brilliance of human intellect, but through the untouchable, unequaled power of the loving God who created us and sustains us through time and all eternity.

Surely the Gospel of Mark could be called the kick butt book of the Bible! It needs to be the kick "but" Gospel too! Read it, receive the message, and refuse to be bound!

Me, Too, and I'll Tell!

When my sister and I were kids, if one of us was sneaking something really good, the other would say, "Me, too, or I'll tell!" Fortunately we don't have to sneak the marvelous, abundant gifts God has for us and when we receive them we need to tell, out loud!

In adult class at church one Sunday, we were studying the councils of the church and the development of the creeds. We discussed the fact of the Trinity being "one" from all time and through all eternity. We also discussed what it meant for Jesus to lay aside His divine powers while in the flesh on earth to show us how we can and should live. If you search the scriptures, you see that He was spared nothing. On the other hand, He was able to perform amazing acts. So often people are very comfortable focusing on the "suffering we share with Jesus" but are very uncomfortable facing the reality of our ability to perform the amazing acts.

Then came the cross, and Jesus freed us from sin and death! He left us with the Holy Spirit, and the ability to do those wonderful things right here, right now. Why are we so much more willing to believe in misery than in victory?

What were those acts? The scripture is full of them. Do your own homework, but just in Mark 3:10-11 we find healing for those who had plagues (diseases) and casting out of unclean spirits. Do you ever encounter people with diseases? Unclean spirits? (Think of people screaming out in alcoholic or drug possession, or unable to speak a sentence without profanity or vulgarity.) There you go.

In 3:15 He gives the disciples the power to heal sicknesses and cast out devils. Yes, they were special people with a special mission, but they and Jesus were working in this world in a physical body of their own, and after Pentecost the power of the Holy Spirit was released to all of us. In the final verse 35, Jesus states clearly, "For whosoever will do the will of God, the same is my brother, and my sister, and my mother." That makes us FAMILY, if we are just willing to do our Father's Will.

Once we can finally admit the wondrously loving will of God for us, we can embrace the glorious acts we are capable of doing through God's grace. We can shout, "Me too, and I'll tell" and shout it from the rooftops all the days of our lives!

Boo-boos and Ouwies

Neither spell-check nor I know how to spell "ouwies!" This word comes from "ouch!" It is the second most popular term for hurts used in childhood, closely following "boo-boo." The cure for them was well known to all kids: hopefully there was some parent or other loving person available who could kiss them and make them feel better.

Then we grow up. Sadly, even little babies may have to face more serious health issues and hurt. Adult diseases, aided and abetted by sin and rebellion, complicate the issue even more, because we forget to run to the loving Father for kisses to make them "all better."

My first skinned knee brought a lesson I've never forgotten. Mother and Daddy kissed it, but then they explained that God would make it well. They prayed to Him, asking for this healing, and then encouraged me to watch my knee every day to see how God would heal it. Guess what! He did! I learned Whom to run to!

One of the most poignant statements in the Bible for me is in Job 42:5, "I have heard of thee by the hearing of the ear, but now my eye sees thee." The personal, intimate, immediate presence of our powerful and loving Heavenly Father was His will for us from the beginning. Genesis tells us that He walked the garden in fellowship with Adam and Eve. When that relationship was right, they didn't need any health care plan!

What's the point? It is that we can move beyond hearing about God, and instead actually hear from Him. Separation from Him was never His idea, or His plan, or His will. We can run to Him with every boo-boo and ouwie life can throw at us, and He will catch us up in His tender mercy and fellowship with us and heal us. He will not fail us: "the compassions of the Lord fail not! They are new every morning! Great is thy faithfulness, O God!" (Lamentations 3:22-23).

If you have never experienced that or have moved away from it, find a quiet space TODAY, and ask the Father to hold you and heal you, to reveal Himself to you in all His love and compassion and tenderness. He is longing, out of His great heart, to do just that! He will be present to you, and put those boo-boos and ouwies so far away that your enemy won't even be able to spell them!

What's the Price?

Used to be (as we southerners say) after the fall, Satan could afflict us with all kinds of diseases that could take us out. This was not God's idea. It came about when man threw away the wonderful disease-free walk in the garden in fellowship with our Heavenly Father 24/7/365. Cast out of that garden, our enemy the deceiver could inflict us with pain and suffering (you could get a backache from pulling those weeds, plowing, planting) and finally he could kill us. How many of us thought as children that we are born, we live, we get sick, AND THEN WE DIE? Probably, all of us!

But then along comes Easter: Resurrection Sunday! We bellow out "Where, O death, is now thy sting?" which is the adult way of taunting: "nah nah nah nah nah!" Not to be sacrilegious, but I'm reminded of the line in that song that goes, "...and then along came Mary!"[3] For us, one day, along came Mary and then along came Jesus and then He paid the price for us in FULL. Every sin, every disease, every infirmity! Not only do we *not* have to get sick and die, but also now we get to live forever with our God just like back in the garden!

So what's the point of sickness and disease? It's still around, isn't it? But it can't take us out because Jesus took it out on the cross. THINK ABOUT IT! YES, I __AM__ SHOUTING!

My mother always remarked in any conversation about eternal life that she was so looking forward to getting there and being able to have all her questions answered. She would always get this dreamy-eyed look on her face like she always got when she was looking for a pencil to start making a list.

For me, the point of that pencil about the enemy's power was broken on the cross, and I have no plans to sharpen it up with doubt. When he tries to throw stuff like FLU on us (and defeated though he is, he never quits trying), I scream, "How DARE you?" and Moe yells, "NO! Not in MY HOUSE!" and shakes the Bible in his face to prove it. After all, since Easter, victory is the only point.

The Workman is Worthy

Check out Matthew 10:7-10. No, I mean really do it! Jesus has equipped His disciples and sent them out. He instructs them to

1) Share the gospel,
2) Heal the sick,
3) Cleanse the lepers,
4) Raise the dead, and
5) Cast out devils. He says, "Freely you have been given, freely give." He also instructs them not to take provisions.

Until today people have quoted this to me insisting that people doing God's work were supposed to be broke! Today the dim bulb lit up and the words "for the workman is worthy of his meat" leaped out at me like fireworks going off in my mind!

The message I get from this is that the workman who is doing God's work will be paid for it. It is GOD, not our smarts, Who gives us the power to perform these amazing acts. It is GOD Who will reward them. Let me ask you this question: do you think those people could have packed for a trip any better than God could reward them for their work? I don't think so! He reminds them, and us, that they have been given freely! With an open hand! With all they could possibly need and more!

If we are not well rewarded now, what could this mean? That God is a cheapskate? That He's out of funds? That He wants His children barely getting by? Worried about money? Sick? Busted and disgusted? OR could it POSSIBLY be that we are not out there doing the work?

How have you been doing lately with sharing the Gospel? Healing, cleansing, raising, and casting out? We can read about it and say "yes, amen" or we can DO IT. Then, God Himself tells us, "the workman is worthy of his meat."

I don't know which is more important for me to consider first, the "workman" part or the "worthy" part, but I'll tell you one thing, this girl has some serious thinking to do. How about you?

Be Prepared

Proverbs 10:22: "The blessing of the Lord makes men rich, and He adds no sorrow to it." "The blessing of the Lord makes men rich; neither shall He add affliction to it."

There are many translations of this scripture. I quoted from King James and Douay-Rheims above. The point in all of them is that God freely gives His beloved children wealth, blessings, goods, riches, but with NO SORROW and with NO AFFLICTION added! Understanding this is huge, especially when the rubber hits the road. If you're not prepared in your own personal, behind-closed-doors faith, you will miss a truth: unlimited power.

By this time you should be convinced that God wants ONLY good, ONLY THE BEST for you. How sad that we have to take time convincing people of that, but we do. How sad that people get "saved" not knowing the fullness of what they can be saved from! With that knowledge (and if you don't know what that means, go back and review all the healing scriptures and messages), we can move forward to the awesome truth:

1) It is GOD who gives us blessings, wealth, and health but 2) WITH NO SORROW added!

Why am I so fired up about this? Because when affliction hits you, it is usually unexpected. It is often a shock! How we react to it in that moment is critical. A sudden slam of affliction should be an immediate tip off that this is NOT from God and it NOT His will and does NOT belong to us.

I'm sorry if that offends anyone, but check it out for yourself. When some awful thing hits me or mine unexpectedly I know immediately that it is not of God and does not belong to me, so I can immediately reject it and flee to the safety and protection and love and POWER of Almighty God.

When you are at this point, you will be amazed that fear does not enter in to the picture at all! We had an example in our lives recently, and the emergency/ ambulance/ ER people were so puzzled that none of us were afraid during some very upsetting circumstances. People kept saying to me, "You're his WIFE?" I guess they were expecting hysteria. I knew that God had it all under control, because He gives me wealth with NO SORROW. If we were dealing with sorrow, it was just junk from the defeated enemy and no big deal. It was already taken care of.

Thank God, the faith was prepared ahead of the need for it. No sorrow can take control. "Thank you, God, I am a VERY wealthy woman! And I have a very healthy husband, thank You very much! In Jesus name, Amen!"

Steadfast and Stand Fast

Lamentations 3:22-24 (RSV): "The steadfast love of the Lord never ceases, **His** mercies never come to an end; they are new every morning; great is thy faithfulness. The Lord is my portion, says my soul, therefore I will hope in Him."

Galatians 5:1: "For freedom Christ has set us free; stand fast therefore, and do not submit again to a yoke of slavery."

What do we do when we pray for healing and it doesn't seem to be working? What do we do when we get healed, and then sickness comes on us again? We focus on the power and will of GOD, not on the problem.

We get stubborn about what God has promised us and refuse to accept anything less, remembering that we are FREE and no longer have to submit to evil or to be vulnerable to it.

The Lord is STEADFAST, so we can be assured that if we will STAND FAST, His mercies will be renewed every morning, available to us without ceasing because of His love for us.

I can remember waiting for HOURS on Route 50 here in Maryland to get across a bridge to the beach in summer. Hours! All of us were determined to get there. I have a friend who waited hours to get a toy her child especially wanted for Christmas. I know people who will wait endlessly for tickets to a concert they want to see. If we can be stubborn in these silly things, certainly we can be stubborn enough to not budge until we get health!

See you at the beach!

The Belt of Truth

I was re-reading Ephesians 6:10-18. Whenever I am tempted to feel a little beaten, a little faint, a little, well, you know, Ephesians and Daniel jerk the slack out of me fast! They are a GREAT antidote for the "poor me" syndrome!

These verses throw all the weapons of our warfare right on the table in front of us and DARE us to arm ourselves and get with the program instead of mumbling and grumbling around.

Ask the Lord to show you your armor in 14-17.

The Belt of Truth is so essential. It keeps us from believing the nonsense the enemy is telling us, what foolish people are telling us, what the media is telling us, what people who love us are telling us, and sometimes what we are telling ourselves. The belt of truth is the divine B.S. detector! Strap it on and get a clear-eyed view of what is REALLY going on.

You may be surprised to learn that the battle you face is different from what you believed.

The Belt Again

Earlier we buckled on the belt of truth. I am hoping that the previous messages, digging out the TRUTH about God's will for our health and healing, has resulted in a simple, irrefutable, and permanent conviction in all our lives now for which this message will be an affirmation.

Jesus promises us that we shall know the truth and the truth shall set us free (John 8:32). How is that working for you? Are you free to receive the facts about how you and yours should be able to walk in health, to expect health, to demand what is your right? If not, does the belt need to be taken in a notch? Or did you leave it hanging in the closet one-day and wind up with the flu?

Was "THE BELT" a threat for discipline for you or anyone you knew growing up? Did you ever hear, "Now you obey me, I don't want to have to get the belt?" On both sides of my family, a belt was hung on a nail for instructional purposes. I am assured that it did not need to be used, or only on the rarest occasion, because the reminder was more than enough to HALT bad behavior.

Our heavenly Father does not threaten us with punishment, or need to "teach us" by inflicting or allowing sickness and disease. NO! Quite the opposite! He gives us the BELT of TRUTH to protect us, and to remind the enemy that his bad behavior will not be tolerated.

Ephesians 6:14 instructs us to keep that belt around our waists, available at all times, for the purpose of that reminder. It reminds us of who we are, whose we are, and our rights in Him. It is a reminder to the enemy/sickness/disease/peril that we are strong in that truth. We have the belt on! So back off, Jack!

If you haven't already done so, get out the belt today. It once hung on a nail on the cross, but now that nail and the cross are empty and you are free!

Full Armor Against What?

As we are, I sincerely expect, putting on the full armor of God in our fight against sickness, disease, and all other "tribulations of this world," we are warned that our fight is not with flesh and blood.

"For our struggle is not against flesh and blood, but against the rulers, against the authorities, against the powers of this dark world and against the spiritual forces of evil in the heavenly realms" (Ephesians 6:11).

It is easy to forget that what we are experiencing is very much in the flesh and blood! The concept in verse 11 may seem hard to understand. We can get distracted by wondering about who these rulers, authorities and powers of this dark world may be and what about the spiritual forces of evil in heavenly realms?

These are good questions! Doing some research here will pay off big time! However the bottom line of immediate importance is to recognize that *the real cause is not in the flesh that is hurting*. We need to jerk our attention away from what we feel and see so that we can focus on the real cause instead of the symptoms. Otherwise we may defeat and exhaust ourselves fighting the physical battle in this playground while our enemy is winning the real battle across the street in the other playground.

If you think about it, the worst part of most illness is often fear, distraction, mental and emotional exhaustion, panic, and unanswered questions. All of these are spiritual, not physical. Think about how it would have been if none of these things had been a part of your last fight with sickness. Wow!

I have been privileged to observe some amazing Christians in my life go through "tribulation." I mean big stuff, without turning a hair. How are they able to do it? They identified the real enemy and the real battle and didn't waste time.

Keeping my armor polished takes work, but I just love to flash it in the eyes of my real enemy when sickness threatens! We've got his number and there's not a thing he can do about it. The sword of the defeated foe is broken before the glorious victory of our risen Lord.

The Breastplate of Righteousness

Have you noticed that in so many scriptures we've referenced concerning healing how often Jesus forgives sins at the same time He heals someone? Matt. 9:2, Luke 5:24, Luke 7:48 are a few examples. Clearly sin is a handicap to healing.

The enemy has twisted the truth (as always) and made people think that they can't receive or don't deserve healing because they are sinners. This is totally unscriptural! Look how Jesus points that out, as He heals people left and right, forgiving them at the same time. He knows that feelings of guilt and unworthiness could rob us of healing, so He deals with that first!

The breastplate of righteousness is an interesting weapon. The breastplate protects the HEART of the soldier. Righteousness will protect OUR hearts too. Doing what is right and refusing evil is powerful protection. Every time we chose to do wrong, we open a "wrong door" that allows evil entry, creating a chink in our armor every time.

Thank goodness God is more faithful than we are. His compassions are new every morning, and great is His faithfulness! If we are sorry and repent then He is faithful to forgive, and His love seals that chink up so that we are not vulnerable in the hole we created.

Don't be deceived by failing to receive your healing because of the knowledge of your own sin. Righteousness is the will of God for you and He will help you find it, cling to it, insist on it, and keep your armor strong and bright. Remember, it protects your heart.

Still Polishing...

"Therefore, there is now no condemnation for those who are in Christ Jesus" (Romans 8:1).

Still hung up on the sin thing? Is that still a potential stumbling block to rob you of the healing grace that is freely given to you if you can just receive it? Take a long, deep, satisfying swig of Romans 8:1 and sober up! Oh yes, getting drunk on the Word is so much more gratifying than the best keg party ever, and there is NO HANGOVER (no sorrow) to follow!

Romans 8 is just the best scripture to rid us of any hang-up of the flesh, which can manifest itself in either sin/condemnation or sickness/disease. The entire flesh deal is NAILED by the indwelling Spirit. Can't you just tell that Paul has truly "been there/done that" and he was so eager to tell us the good news so we can get free too?

Check out verse 11: "But if the Spirit of Him that raised up Jesus from the dead dwells in you, He that raised up Christ from the dead shall also quicken your mortal bodies by His Spirit that dwells in you."

I love the way this verse focuses squarely on the right here, right now. In heaven we won't have to deal with sin or sickness, will we? Our mortal bodies will have ceased to be an issue. No, this promise is for us here in the flesh, and it is the best news a healing team could hear.

Once we accept that, life in the flesh is transformed. We can put on that breastplate of righteousness with no doubt, no hesitation, no condemnation, fully convinced that we are fully deserving, not because of what we could ever do but because of what He did for us!

Get Your Shoes On!

One last note on Ephesians 6:14 regarding the breastplate of righteousness: once in a rather heated conversation with my mother about doing the right thing (that I did NOT want to do), I flipped out. I said, "I know, Mom, it is necessary to do right. However, it is NOT necessary to be happy!" to which she immediately replied, "Right!" We both laughed then, and in a calmer frame of mind she explained that if we choose to happily do wrong, all our protection is removed one bit at a time, and we will become very miserable very quickly.

Now, on to verse 15: "...with your feet fitted with the readiness that comes from the gospel of peace." The good news that brings peace is really the beginning of any kind of healing. The realization that this pain and suffering and FEAR is not the will of God and you don't have to accept it and put up with it is huge. But what's this about the feet fitted with readiness?

I am not a theologian, which you've no doubt figured out by now, but God is doing a work in me about this. Think about putting shoes on for some serious travel. I am not a runner/jogger, but those of you who are definitely pay attention to the shoes you wear, don't you? Those shoes are critical to the success of the undertaking, no doubt about it. Ditto for golf shoes, cleats, and ballet slippers. You get the idea.

I relate in the arena of SHOPPING! Let me tell you, when I get ready for MY recreational sport/art I pay serious attention to the shoes I wear. I can hear the "Amen, Sister!" from all the ladies out there!

Just putting on the right shoes is key to READINESS, the readiness that comes from the good news. That readiness is the "shoe" the gospel of peace has prepared for us, the most important and exciting and critical shoe any of us will ever wear. The kicker is, we have to put the shoes on ourselves.

I am suppressing the desire to run over to DSW right now! I am already wearing the most priceless footwear, and my feet are indeed ready to take the gospel of peace throughout the world, shopping for souls paid for by the price of the cross.

Extinguishing Flaming Arrows

"In addition to all this, take up the shield of faith, with which you can extinguish all the flaming arrows of the evil one" Ephesians 6:16.

People who don't know or believe that the scripture is true must have an awful time getting through life with all the flaming arrows the enemy is shooting at us all day every day. What a terrible way to live and how unnecessary! In this case, ignorance is not bliss; it's terror and worry and suffering.

None of us have any business being in that category, even for a second. This scripture has a powerful promise: we can EXTINGUISH those fiery arrows, ALL of them! We can blow them out like the frail little candles on a birthday cake because our enemy aiming them at us is a frail little defeated foe, unable to penetrate our SHIELD of FAITH.

Did you ever get a cake with those trick candles that you can't blow out? God does not work like that. He does not tease us. He gives us a weapon that cannot be penetrated as a GIFT.

Faith is a gift of the Holy Spirit (I Cor. 12), so that shield is not something we have to work up ourselves! It belongs to you for your protection against ANY "arrow" of the evil one. You do, however, have to accept that gift, and pick it up, and use it as a shield instead of running around carrying on.

Be assured that this promise is true. Open up your gift, take up your shield of faith, and you'll be fully able to blow out all the flaming arrows with one puff!

The Helmet

The scripture verses included at the end of this message will focus our thinking on...our thinking! If we are strong, victorious, overcoming Christians we need to think like grownups, and accept that what we REALLY think reveals who we REALLY are. Human imagination since the fall is easily inclined toward evil...but thanks be to God, what GOD imagines for us and thinks about us is too marvelous for us to even dream or imagine!

The Helmet of Salvation protects our thoughts, minds, words, and decisions from the evil inclinations of fallen man. Salvation means we are redeemed from wrong thinking and are free from the trap. However, we must keep that helmet firmly on our heads to protect our thinking from all the false information that bombards us every day from every direction.

For a "healing example," we can't afford to listen to people, read articles about or overhear lengthy discussion about all the various tales of sickness and disease! WALK AWAY from these murmurings! BE CAREFUL about what you allow to enter your mind. Is what you are hearing or seeing TRUE enough to penetrate the Helmet of Salvation? If not, WALK AWAY. Refuse to allow your mind to be polluted!

The most dangerous sources are those dear loving friends or family who want to sympathize with you or others who are encountering illness or injury, forever focusing on, asking about, and sharing similar stories about the suffering. Unless you know the person you are around is a strong believer, avoid any discussion on this topic. They don't have to know! You can be fully convicted of God's will for healing, and some sweet soul can steal it away from you with the very best intentions.

I have found that as a general rule, the best policy is to just SHUT UP!!! Refuse to advertise Satan's work in the world! No matter what, you can always say, "I'm believing for a great outcome!" Then stop it right there. You can tell people in recovery how much better they look and sound! You ladies can throw on some lipstick and a smile even if you feel like an irritated dishrag. You men can shave and grin and insist on demanding a good report!

Why? Because our goal is to think like Jesus, who never concentrated on or talked about the illness or infirmity or death (look it up) but just quietly took care of it with His faith-filled words and His love. Yes I know we are not Jesus, but we can learn to THINK like Him, and to keep that helmet on so that nothing contradictory to His thoughts is allowed to influence us.

Good news! The helmet is a one -size-fits-all deal. It fits hard heads, soft heads, sleepyheads, rockheads, big heads. Yep, it fits all of us! It makes football and motorcycle helmets look like Barbie toys by comparison. Keep your helmet handy, and don't leave home without it!

1 Corinthians 14:20

Brethren, do not be children in your thinking; be babes in evil, but in thinking be mature**.**

Proverbs 23:7

...for as He thinketh in His heart**,** so is he**.**

Genesis 6:5

The Lord saw how great the wickedness of the human race had become on the earth, and that every inclination of the thoughts of the human heart was only evil all the time.

Proverbs12:20

Deceit is in the heart of them that imagine evil, but to the counselors of peace there is joy.

Ephesians 3:20-21

Now to Him who is able to do immeasurably more than all we ask or imagine, according to His power that is at work within us, to Him be glory in the church and in Christ Jesus throughout all generations, for ever and ever! Amen.

Association Caution!

The Helmet of Salvation is a powerful protection for our minds... IF we put it on, and IF it does not slip off.

How could it happen that we wouldn't put it on? Have you put yours on today? Or did you forget all about it until you started reading this? (Can't you hear your enemy saying right now, "Oh NUTS!"?) Put it on right now, and then continue.

That helmet and all the other weapons are free gifts from God (the price was paid in full, remember?) but WE must choose to receive and use them.

OK, you have it on. Can it slip? Yes, in many ways: distraction, anger, sin...the list goes on. One big caution that I'd like to mention is the words and influence of other people.

You are probably surrounded in your daily life by people who are believing and speaking things about sickness, disease, injury, and any number of things in a way that DO NOT LINE UP with what the Word of God says. DANGER! CAUTION!

Be careful, because just by hearing these things from kindly, sincere, well intentioned people, your healing or health can be stolen from you. Because they ARE kindly, sincere, well intentioned, and ignorant of God's will, you can listen politely and be influenced. Feel the helmet slipping?

Inquiries or sympathy can be deadly if they distract your focus from your faith. What should we do in these situations? We may say, "Thank you for caring, but I'm believing for 100% recovery, or 100% health." To a Christian believer (and sadly so many Christians are unaware of God's will for health) we might say, "Thanks so much, but I need prayers of praise for 100% healing, because that's what the scripture tells me to expect." If all else fails, it is critical to WALK AWAY.

Even overhearing the long litanies about how bad poor so and so is doing can affect your thoughts. Move to another table, take a different seat on the bus, collect the dishes and escape to the kitchen!

Most of all, know the people you can trust. I thank God profusely that I have a husband and some friends who absolutely refuse to accept or dwell on or pay attention to the attacks/fiery arrows/tribulations! When they encounter trouble, they immediately go into their own attack mode: "I speak LIFE to you," they say. "No weapon formed against you shall prosper!" they remind us. "By His stripes you are healed!" they insist. Praise God for people who know the truth when the chips are down!

Do you know people you can count on like this? If not, find some fast! They'll help you keep your helmet on.

> *Heavenly Father, we thank you so much for those faithful people in our lives, and ask that you help us to find more. Help us to become that kind of person ourselves! Thank you for the weapons of our warfare. We pray that through the Holy Spirit we may learn more and grow stronger in the truth every day, so that our minds are the mind of Christ, our words in 100% agreement with your Word, and our lives a strong and beautiful example to a world so in need of both the knowledge and the experience of your wonderful strength and love. In Jesus name, Amen*

Permanent Promises

"Jesus Christ the same yesterday, today, and forever!" Hebrews 3:8

Some of us get it; some of us long for it, but the glorious truth of this scripture one day breaks through to us and stuns us with its power. He has not changed. What He did for others, He will do for us! What He did on earth in human flesh, WE CAN DO on earth in human flesh! Glory!

Do not be afraid to accept biblical promises—you can trust your Heavenly Father. When you open His gifts, they are as wonderful for you as they were for those who were healed by Jesus. Healing is absolutely a gift of the Holy Spirit, ready to abide and work in you both for yourself and for others.

In order to be saved and assured of everlasting life you had to believe that God loved you and would forgive your sins. In order to walk in health you have to believe that God loves you and will heal your body. Scripture states bluntly that, "As many (sinners) who received Him were born of God." (I John 1:12-13) AND as many sick who "touched Him were made whole." (Mark 6:56)

Even death is not fearful for us. We know it is just a translation into everlasting life. Have you ever heard anyone say, "I don't mind being dead but I don't like the thought of dying." What good news for them to learn that you don't have to be sick to die! You can just close your eyes and go home!

Ps. 104:29: "You take away their breath, they die and return to their dust."

Job 5:26: "You shall come to your grave in a full age, like as a shock of corn comes in its season."

Psalm 92:14: after having lived a fruitful life...

Exodus 23:26: fulfilling the number of your days...

I Thess. 4:17: So shall you ever be with the Lord!

This is the blessed hope of the righteous.

It is a permanent promise that does not change or go away for all of us who will accept it.

"Because you have set your love upon me", God tells us, "therefore I will deliver you: I will set you on high, because you have known my name. You shall call upon me and I will answer you; I will be with you in trouble; I will deliver you and honor you. With long life I will satisfy you, and show you my salvation." (Psalm 91:14-16)

We receive this, Lord! Thank you!"

Hungry for Healing

Women who are pregnant for the first time—and their husbands—are often astonished at the sudden and powerful hunger that overtakes these mothers to be. They have to eat RIGHT NOW! My friend Judy shared this story: "Steve and I were traveling to visit relatives in another state. All of a sudden I said to Steve, "I have to eat, and I have to eat right now. Pull over at the very next place that has any kind of food. Whatever they're cooking, that's what I'm having!"

When we have that kind of hunger for the Word, we can begin to learn all we need to know about healing, or any other need in our lives. God reassures us that our hunger will be satisfied. For example, in Luke 6:21, "Blessed are you that hunger now, for you will be filled." Those words were spoken to people who had traveled great distances on foot to hear His teaching and to receive His healing (6:17). They were hungry for information and for healing, and they got them!

What often happens, however, is that unless we are hurting or ailing we may not feel hungry. We may ignore the information and health that is available to us until disaster hits. When it does hit, we may be like Judy, ready to eat/receive the first thing that comes along, and that can be dangerous. Be warned! Just ANY information can be wrong, harmful or waste valuable, maybe critical, time.

We must be hungry for God's Word, for vital information, BEFORE a crisis hits. If we do, when it does we are ready. There is no panic, fear, doubt, or hand wringing! We KNOW what to do, because we have been filled.

I pray for us today that all of us will be as ravenously hungry as a pregnant woman for the Word and yes, you guys too! Let us seek the Lord who promises us all the information and the healing we will ever need and assures us that we will be filled.

Stubborn Determination from II Kings 4

I found a passage I had loved and lost. Now I have it and can share it with you. So this day must be the appointed day for all of us to rejoice over it!

It concerns a Shunammite woman. (How I wish I knew her name!) In II Kings 4:19 the woman's son goes to his father crying, "My head, my head!" He is taken to his mother, who holds him until noon, and then he dies. She immediately takes him to the bed in the guest room where the prophet Elisha stays when he visits. She closes the door and leaves.

She asks her husband to get the car ready. (Ok, so it was one of the asses, but those were their means of transportation.) She asks him to get it ready because she is going to the prophet. She does not tell him or anyone else that the boy is dead. She just says, "All will be well." She travels quite a distance, and when she is near Elisha's house his servant Gehazi runs to greet her and asks how the family is doing, and she says "It is well." Can you believe that? It is well!

When she finally reaches Elisha, she tells him what has happened, and he instructs Gehazi to go and lay his staff on the boy. Gehazi takes off, but the Shunammite woman tells Elisha she is not leaving until Elisha comes with her. He has the sense not to argue with her, and he goes. Even a tough man knows better than to mess with a mother protecting her young.

When Gehazi goes in to the boy and lays the staff on him, nothing happens. He reports this to Elisha as he approaches the house. So Elisha goes in and, well, you have to read this for yourself. Verses 34-37 touch me deeply. How I wish I'd had this knowledge when my son Gabriel died.

The woman got what she had spoken out of her mouth! She got what she insisted upon! This woman had faith that would not let go. She refused to speak what she did not want to her husband, to her household, and to Gehazi. She refused to compromise, too. How right she was, because Gehazi was not up to the job. It had to be Elisha! Elisha knew better than to argue with her, didn't he?

That's my kind of woman and my kind of faith! I want to walk in that kind of conviction all the days of my life. I want to know my rights and my authority and to be a real pain in the you-know-what until that faith is manifested! Clearly her husband did not yet have that faith, so she could not tell him when the boy died. My Moe DOES have that kind of faith, so he and I can stubbornly stand together. But isn't it comforting to know that you can have it all by yourself, and your faith will be sufficient? It's not you, it's God who will honor stubborn determination!

So, let's review the two lessons here: 1) Be careful whom you tell, and 2) Be a real pain in the you-know-what, until you get it! (The gospel lesson according to Sharon!)

Slap Yourself, and Pay Attention!

Are you or any of your loved ones or people on your prayer list continually ailing with something? Go look in the mirror for a possible reason. Or as my dear friend, Joanne, would say, "Slap yourself!"

Of course, it may not be your fault that you, or they, got that way, but you certainly should have something to do with getting them healed. I do not include people who refuse healing. Sometimes people resist it, and some receive it and then let it go. This is not your fault, unless you are the culprit doing yourself in or talking someone else out of their healing.

This is not intentional! It can happen the way some people don't read text or email messages promptly and miss out on important information. If you are ignoring the scripture, failing to seek wisdom to strengthen your faith and power, you can become ineffective just by failing to pay attention.

If that's you, wake up! "He who has ears, let him hear" (Matthew 11:15). Get the power! Pay attention! Even if you have to slap yourself!

Turn Can't Into Can

Zechariah 4:6
"Then He said to me, This is the word of the Lord to Zerub'babel: Not by might, nor by power, but by my Spirit, says the Lord of hosts."

II Corinthians 12:9
"My grace is sufficient for you, for my power is made perfect in weakness."

Sometimes we may be tempted to feel that we just don't have the strength or the power to overcome, even by faith, the attacks against us in our bodies or our minds. Whether this feeling comes as the result of exhaustion, pain, or stress, we may reach a point where we are tempted to conclude, "I just can't do it."

This is the door to doubt and discouragement at best and to suicide at worst. Know this, it is the SAME DOOR! So beware, you certainly should know better than to open it. It you didn't know before, you know right now. Do you sense a "Because I said so!" coming from me? I am not your parent, and it is not because I said so anyway, it is because God said so.

If you have done your best to walk in faith, and refuse to be tempted by the world, the flesh, and the devil and just feel worn down, be of good cheer! Jesus has overcome the world, the flesh and the devil!

The feeling of "I can't" is partially accurate; after all, we can't take our next breath without God. We can't control gravity or keep the planets in place, not without the power of God. We don't have the might or the power or the authority to do any of that.

However, God does, and we are His, and His strength and power surround us all the time. He promises to dwell in us. His power takes care of our breath, gravity, the planets, and everything else! WE don't have to be mighty and powerful because He is mighty and powerful, and by His Spirit we can participate in the safety of that power (Zech. 4:6).

Naturally, compared to God we are weak, but with God, we are invincible! Whimpering, "Oh I just can't do this…" is really a sign of pride rather than humility, because it suggests that we can handle all the other stuff of daily life by ourselves. Think about it.

The truth is we can't do squat without Him and we can do everything with Him. Between you and God, there is absolutely nothing you can't accomplish. Sorry Sweetheart, but that excuse is now gone forever. In our weakness God steps in, and at our invitation takes over and accomplishes whatever needs to get done. His grace trumps your weakness every time (II Cor. 12:9)!

So get out there and don't worry about your shabby little weaknesses! Tell them who you are! When they ask, "Who do you think you are?" let them see that you are a child of the Living God, the greatest power in the universe! Turn your "can't" into "can" starting today!

Quality Control

What is it that keeps us from possessing health, or any of the other blessings God offers us so freely; that Jesus has won for us on the cross? Like most stumbling blocks, this is often a simple issue of control. We want what we want when we want it, we want to do things OUR way and so we fail to receive the far greater riches (with NO SORROW) that would be ours if we'd just choose God's way.

Scripture assures us that God's goodness is only limited by our capacity to receive it. It is clear in His Word (both in scripture and in the person of Jesus, the Living Word) about the rules/laws we must follow for our own protection. The Ten Commandments are pretty blunt: put God first, have no other gods, honor His Name, keep the Sabbath holy, honor your parents, don't murder, kill, commit adultery, steal, lie, or go after (even in imagination!) what does not belong to you. As Moe says, "This is so simple, you have to have help to misunderstand it!" Of course, the enemy is always all too ready to do that job.

"Blessed is the man", says Psalm 12, "who fears the Lord and delights greatly in His <u>commandments</u>..." That psalm reminds us that wealth and riches will overtake us as well! So many people are afraid to receive what God has for us. Not I! I want to receive every single thing my Father has for me! II Chronicles 25:9 tells me "...the Lord is able to give you much more than this." Wow, no matter what I receive there is still much more! Sign me up for much more than this right now!

Instead of exercising our own control over everything, and accepting far less than the very best, why not exercise quality control and insist on the best, God's best for our lives. When we do that with no reservation, we will be BOLD in demanding nothing less. Proverbs 28:1 nails it: "The wicked flee when no man pursues, but the righteous are bold as a lion."

Who are the righteous? Those who obey the commandments, walk in God's ways, and accept nothing less than His best. How do you stack up? Get with the program and exercise some quality control today!

Ticket to Ride

Because of an upcoming function I had the fun of creating some tickets yesterday...and of course that got me thinking about the significance of tickets. Life is a journey for each of us, and where we wind up will be determined by the "tickets to ride" that we select. They will move us to health, strength, "nothing missing, nothing broken," or to sickness, weakness and a total train wreck! We must decide first where we want to go, and then choose the tickets that will take us there.

The Ten Commandments and many other guidelines in scripture teach us clearly the physical acts to perform or avoid. The deeper impact of right or wrong choices, and the underlying reality exposed about us in the choices we make, manifests itself in the result. Have you read those statistics indicating that a vast percentage of people in hospitals are there because of a spiritual issue that eventually lead to a physical manifestation in the body?

Think about the unhealthy doors, from a medical perspective, that adultery opens. It begins with a spiritual detour in the imagination that finally leads to a physical act having serious consequences. Physical, emotional, and mental disorders all have a source, a ticket someone selected to ride with disastrous consequences for himself and/or others.

Honoring false gods and dishonoring the name of God lead to hideous consequences, even something as simple as failure to keep the Sabbath holy. I am stunned by the number of nice people I know who have no regard for the Sabbath. How many even ask a blessing over their food? The final destination will reflect those choices.

We need to carefully, prayerfully select the tickets to ride, because they will inevitably take us one direction or another. Want your loved ones to be healthy and safe? Pay more attention to what you model and teach spiritually than to what you do physically. Show them the tickets to ride to safe places, where they can live in peace, health, and all the blessings in the right destinations.

Decide where you want to go, and then choose the ticket that will take you there.

Do Some Yelling!

John 16:33: "These things I have spoken to you so that you might have peace. In the world you shall have tribulation: but be of good cheer: I have overcome the world."

This word is so blunt and clear and to the point, how can we possibly miss it? Jesus did what He did so we could have PEACE. He says THE WORLD will have tribulation, but that's not for us. Yes it will come toward us...but He has already overcome it for us!

Sickness, disease, accidents, misfortunes, sorrow, pain, betrayal—they'll come at us in the world, but we don't have to take them out to lunch! This is what you need to say to all the junk that tries to trap you, "YOU DO NOT BELONG TO ME." They say that using caps means you're yelling, and that's what we need to do! Yell the truth in the enemy's face. Have you done any yelling lately? Or have you just been whispering in quiet desperation?

Get with the program! How? I remember the song:

Turn your eyes upon Jesus
Look full in His wonderful face,
And the things of this world will grow strangely dim
In the light of His glory and grace.
(Helen H. Lemmel 1922 Public Domain)[4]

We cannot afford to let our eyes drift from Him. When we keep His marvelous face before us, we know that we have absolutely NOTHING to fear or to worry about.

Do some yelling today!

It's Who You Know

"Beloved, I wish in all things that you may prosper and be in good health, even as your soul prospers." (3 John 2)

The word "health" in this scripture comes from a Greek word *hugiaino*, which means healthy, sound, free from disease, or free from germs that could cause sickness and disability. No, I do not speak Greek. I depend on my friends who do in moments like these; sometimes it's not what you know but who you know!

Isn't it shocking how easily most people are firmly convinced that sickness, disability, debt, poverty, and lack are just normal parts of life, and so they accept them? This is the will of Satan, yet they are reluctant to trust in the promises of God, who offers life and health and prosperity and all good things. Think about the people you know. Think about yourself.

The story for this scripture is about the plans John and his group of ministers had to visit the church of a man named Gaius. This man was literally worrying himself sick because a wealthy and influential man in the church, Diotrephes, did not want this visit and threatened to cut off financial support if they came. Don't you love it that the scripture names names? After all these centuries, the story of these two men, the personal story, comes down to us in a very personal way! Men like these are everywhere in our own culture!

However, Gaius knew John. John points out that Diotrephes: 1) does not have a corner on all the money in the world, and 2) is kicking sand because he likes to be in control. He reminds Gaius that GOD is his source, and wants to be his source of supply. Let's face it, God has always had way more money than Diotrephes, the Astors, Vanderbilts, Soros, Gates or anyone else!

For heaven's sake, we can count on God for everything, including *hugiaino*, even if we don't speak Greek. John assures his friend that he is praying that he will prosper and be in good health, even as his soul prospers. We are reading it today. You need to write in the margin, "I, too, will prosper and be in good health, even as my soul prospers!"

Our resources and our health can be placed with total faith in the hands of our Heavenly Father, who has the corner on every source of supply. We know Him! It's not what you know, but Who you know!

Healing, Conditional Promises

"If you abide in me, and my words abide in you, you shall ask whatever you will and it shall be done to you." (John 15:7)

God's love for us is unconditional. Nothing we can do will cause Him to love us less or to love us more. However, healing and other blessings are not unconditional. They are "If/then" promises, which means we must take action in order to receive them. This passage from John 15 is one of these types of promises.

Let's say you are longing and praying for healing. You won't get it just hoping and carrying on crying and pleading. You will get it when you pay attention to the "if" part of this conditional promise. God instructs us that we must abide in Him, and that His word must abide in us before that prayer can be answered.

Recently I have spent a great deal of time considering the Word as Jesus in the flesh ("...and the Word became flesh and dwelt among us"). In my own flesh, I can absolutely tell you that when I am in the presence of God and filled with the scriptures I have been reading, NOTHING else matters. Everything else going on in my flesh or in my life fades to insignificance: pain, sorrow, fear, doubt, stress, irritation, and general cussedness.

God promises us that when we are in that marvelous place, we will receive what we ask. Do you know what's particularly cool about that? When we are in that place, we will never ask anything that is not in accordance with His will! His glory and tenderness are just too wonderful.

Let me give a personal example. By nature, I am not good with details. I get overwhelmed with detailed tasks, especially if many are important at the same time. Yet, in the life to which God has called me, I am constantly swimming in detail work. This can make me stressed, irritable, exhausted, and if I don't get a grip, it can make me ill. However, in the last 24 hours, with one of those lists going down, I was so joyful and energized that I got a TON of stuff done, even the extras! I polished a piece of furniture for no reason at all!

Why? Because I have been working recently on a major project with the Lord that has immersed me in scripture and in conversation with Him. I go to sleep and wake up hearing His voice and hearing scripture. It's the most amazing thing! This scripture is a living word in my life today, and what a feeling!

When you are seeking something really important for your health or anything else, or even some dumb little thing (nothing is too big or too small for our Abba Father), be assured that God will always keep His part of that promise, but you must also keep yours.

Have you ever taught a little child how to tie his or her shoe? You tell him or her and then you show him or her and then in one glorious moment, the child does it. I think the joy of that moment, both for the adult and for the child, must be something like what God feels when we get things like this right!

Healing: Claim Your Benefits!

There has been a lot of discussion in the news recently about "benefits." You know, people looking at job opportunities check carefully into the benefit packages that come along (sometimes) with the job. Given recent changes in the laws and health care, the cost of health benefits for employees has become a financial burden some employers can no longer sustain. Many employers must either stop offering these benefits or employ fewer people.

God offers a very different benefit plan:

"Bless the Lord, O my soul: and all that is within me bless His holy name. Bless the Lord, and forget not all His benefits:
He forgives all your iniquities;
He heals all your diseases:
He redeems your life from destruction..." Psalm 103:1-4

God is not our employer, although He does want us to work with Him! He is our Heavenly Father, so we get extra, such as: "...He crowns you with loving-kindness and tender mercies..." Has any employer ever offered you a package like that?

When you receive benefits through work, they do cost you something. Various health related security benefits available to citizens of the USA are also paid for by citizens of the USA. A bit is taken from your paycheck. Do you remember getting the first paycheck from your first "real" job, and being shocked to see that you didn't actually get the cash you were expecting? What a reality check THAT rite of passage is!

God's benefits, on the other hand, are FREE for you and me. Jesus paid them in full on the cross. Think about that. He took on Himself all the pain, agony, and suffering, and conquered it. Do you think He wasn't up to the job, didn't quite get it done, and needs us to suffer a little more to finish what He wasn't able to accomplish? Absolutely, not!

Why then do some people fail to accept and live in the blessings of God's benefit package? A primary reason is that most people <u>don't</u>

even know about it. Another reason is that many who have read or heard about it don't understand it for what it is. A final reason is that many who understand it are afraid to believe it, receive it and count on it.

Isn't that the craziest thing? That any of us would trust an employer's offer more than we would trust God's?

May I make a modest suggestion here? TAKE THE PACKAGE. Claim your benefits! God NEVER runs out of money, or healing power, or loving kindness. He never lays anybody off because He runs out of money, either!

Go ahead and TRUST Him as your source and your resource. Claim your benefit package today!

No Lists, No Arguments, Just Thanksgiving and Praise!

Recently I was reading a book in which the author mentioned that it is foolish to tell God what we need because He already knows (Matthew 6:8). They also said it was foolish to try to get Him to change His mind. (God never changes. "I am the Lord thy God; I change not." Malachi 3:6.)

Is that what you do when you pray? I'll bet at one time we all fell into that useless behavior because that's all we knew to do. However, now we know better.

God does not change His mind, and He is very clear about His will. He wants us well! We don't have to list for Him all the "tribulations" we encounter, and we don't have to convince Him to help us. We must simply agree with His will in faith, receive our healing, and praise Him for His faithfulness to us.

If we are shaky in our own faith, we may have doubts about God's faithfulness toward us. Think about this: it is interesting how often people believe that other people think just as they do. For instance, a thief is convinced that other people will steal from him. A liar believes that everyone tells lies. These people may not be able to trust even the reliably trustworthy people around them because they are projecting their own character onto others.

Our enemy wants us to do this with God. If he can get someone to doubt God's healing grace and power, he can steal their ability to receive health from their loving Father. We know better!

So if we don't have to list all our needs and worries for God, and we don't have to convince Him to be good to us...what do we pray? Some prayer closets may get mighty quiet here! We can remind Him of His wonderful promises, and praise Him for His perfect will in our lives.

I am so thrilled that God wants you and me well! I rejoice that He wants that even more than we do. I am so grateful that He knows every single need we have even before we know it, and that He has the fulfillment of that need ready to pour out on us. I am so glad we do not need to waste time trying to convince Him to provide the blessings of health, or any other good thing for us. I rejoice in the fact that His wonderful will for us is more than we could ever dream or imagine.

When we are really looking at the bottom line, two words can almost say it all. They are "Thank You!"

Healing, in the Flesh

It takes a lifetime to comprehend that time, including our time here on earth, is a part of eternity. How many times the remembrance of that reality can slip our consciousness, as day-to-day responsibilities occupy our thoughts. Day to day is as important as forever, because it is a part of forever.

This is one reason why I find scripture so amazing. It is filled with messages and information about eternity, but also about the right here, right now, in the physical bodies we occupy. Since our victory over sickness and disease and the other distresses that pertain to our time in the flesh is of here and now importance, finding and meditating on the scriptures about these specific concerns is key.

Consider Proverbs 4:20-22: "My son, attend to my words: incline your ear to my sayings. Do not let them depart from your eyes; keep them in the midst of your heart. For they are life to all those who find them, and health to all their flesh."

When we depart from our flesh, one set of considerations that we must deal with in this temporary life will no longer concern us. However, while we're here they certainly do! How wonderful that God has given us the key right here in this passage: His Word is health to our flesh.

I understand that the Hebrew word for "health" here means "medicine." God's word is medicine for our flesh. That is good news! This medicine is freely available to us, with no medical expense at all. No health plan, insurance, appointments, waiting around, filling out forms, freezing your backside in those little inadequate gowns, tests, scary stuff, nasty medicine, procedures, or side effects!

Such a simple truth, so easily available and freely given: if we pay attention to God's Word, it is medicine and health to our flesh, right here, right now.

"Lord, we are paying attention today! Thank you for always paying attention to us, and providing for all of our needs, both in this life and the next, out of your infinite love."

Healing, Antiseptic for Filthy Dreamers

We are so aware, thanks to advertising and to Granny's admonitions, that the germs which hang out in dirt and filth can hurt us and need to be avoided when possible and scrubbed away when not. "Wash your hands!" we are warned in many circumstances. Recently we are urged to wash long enough to sing "Happy Birthday" before rinsing, so fitting since birthdays celebrate life and so does cleanliness!

However, God warns us also of the danger of dirt in our minds. Our imaginations can be a hotbed of filth and disease far more dangerous than material germs. In the Epistle of Jude, Paul warns us of the inevitable danger for "filthy dreamers." That description really gripped me the first time I read it! "Filthy dreamers," can't you just get a mental picture of these people? If not, turn on late night TV for a few seconds, or listen to the lyrics of a hit song or two on a secular station. Filth is promoted everywhere you turn, readily available to all ages on the home computer, the cell phone, and everywhere else.

I urge you to read Jude, the very short book in the Bible, barely more than a page in length. The actions of these ungodly people began in their imaginations. That's exactly where all of our acts begin. Eventually, we will all act on the things we have repeatedly imagined. The results are inevitable and will lead to sin, sickness, and death.

There's good news! Philippians 4:8 has the antidote: "Finally brothers, whatsoever things are true, whatsoever things are honest, whatsoever things are just, whatsoever things are pure, whatsoever things are lovely, whatsoever things are of good report; if there be any virtue and if there be any praise, think on these things."

Verse 9 has a promise: "Those things which you have both learned and received and heard and seen me do, DO, and the God of peace shall be with you."

DO! Don't you love it? How much simpler can the message be? These verses are a guaranteed antiseptic for filthy dreams. Spray them in your heart and mind today. Kill the germ before it can grow into a stronghold in your flesh! It's probably the most critical health measure/disease prevention we can choose.

Are You in the Right Line?

"A good man brings good things out of the good stored up in his heart, and an evil man brings evil things out of the evil stored up in His heart. For the mouth speaks what the heart is full of." (Luke 6:45)

"What I feared has come upon me; what I dreaded has happened to me." (Job 3:25)

Psalm 23, which most of us memorized as children claims, "I will fear no evil, for thou art with me."

So, how are you doing with fearing no evil? I am not suggesting that you are evil. However, I am suggesting that we need to listen to ourselves and to take our pulse frequently when it comes to fear.

Job and his family were fine—more than fine. However, he began to fear concerning the behavior of his sons. He imagined it, thought about it, and then feared it. When he went before the Lord in worship, he even sacrificed against it. Guess what? The thing he feared most eventually happened, opening the door for Satan's intervention in his life. For what we can gather from scripture here, neither God nor the sons had dreamed up this evil. So guess who was behind it all along?

What does this have to do with healing? Plenty. If we are imagining sickness, disease, infirmity, or other calamity we are in trouble, and we are also in control. We COULD be imagining perfect health, couldn't we? What we imagine will become what we think... will become what we speak ...will determine what will eventually come upon us.

God is always thinking health for us! Satan is always thinking illness for us. Are we going to line up our own thinking with our Father or with our enemy?

Here's a good test: check the words coming out of your mouth, then your thoughts and imagination. How do they line up? Fear is another great test, a sure sign that something you are experiencing or thinking is NOT lining up with the wonderful will of God.

We need for our imaginations, our thoughts, and our words to line up with God. Which line are you in right now? Do you need to make a switch? If so, get in the right line today!

Healing, No Evil; No Fear

"And the Lord shall deliver me from every evil work, and will preserve me unto His heavenly kingdom: to whom be glory forever and ever." (II Timothy 4:18)

"For God has not given us the spirit of fear; but of power, and of love, and of a sound mind." (II Timothy 1:7)

Tent making was such a quiet, peaceful profession. Paul had no idea what he was in for when after his encounter with God not only his name but his whole life would be transformed as he undertook a new calling to serve God in sharing the gospel. At one point he went back to tent making for a time, and I don't blame him! Everybody needs a break when they've faced so many adventures and challenges. In spite of all he had endured when he wrote this letter of encouragement to Timothy, the two scriptures above tell it all, don't they?

No matter what you have endured, in your health adventure or any other, what a wonderful assurance it is to know that God Himself will deliver you from EVERY EVIL WORK, and that He will give you power, love and a sound mind in place of fear.

Just knowing that gives us such an edge. Evil works don't mess with us for long! And we are no longer captives of fear. Think about it: you have power, love, and a sound mind from your heavenly father. Through His mercy, you are well equipped, like Paul, to fight the good fight, being fully assured that you will win.

Thank You!

"For I know whom I have believed, and am persuaded that He is able to keep that which I have committed unto Him against that day" (II Timothy 1:12).

"Give thanks to the Lord for He is good! His merciful kindness endures forever!" (Psalm 118:29)

At a very young age we have to be trained to say "Thank you!" Those are the "magic words" our parents teach us, to combat the tendency for adorable children to take the blessings heaped upon them for granted. As we grow older, those of us who have taken gratitude into our hearts and spirits have a tremendous edge.

When we wake up in the morning, we are so healthy. Yes, I know we may be dealing with some "tribulations," but did you ever make a list of those you DO NOT HAVE, and rejoice over them? Do we get so caught up in the "ouch" that we neglect to thrill on all the glories?

It is so wonderful to praise God and thank Him, not with a list of blessings we've asked for and received, but also with a list of everything that—thanks to Him—we have NOT received!

"Thank you, Lord, for all the arrows that have NOT hit us, all the holes we have stepped over, all the viruses that died right on our surface because of your great indwelling power. Thank you! We praise you for your eternal loving-kindness and the well-being that surrounds us every day because of your powerful love!"

Healing—Ask God First

We have a cute ad on TV in our area for a local car dealership. The general theme is, "Jack says yes!" The viewer is encouraged to check with Jack's dealership first, because he always says "Yes" to whatever you are looking for. You might as well save your time shopping around, it claims, because Jack will say "Yes" to what you want right away!

Isn't it amazing how God is often way down on the list of sources people consult when a health issue or crisis manifests? People spend hours, weeks, months, or sometimes years checking every other source. If something works, fine! If it doesn't, they worry and fret and stress until finally in desperation they turn to God, often approaching Him with "If you're really there God...," pleading for help, "I've tried everything else..."

Jack says "Yes" because he owns the company! He has the authority to give you the car you want, with the bells and whistles you want, in the color you want, at the price you want. God says "Yes" because He owns the universe and He loves you! He will let you know exactly what you need to do to get all your needs fulfilled, including healing!

Let's be cautious that we don't have more faith in Jack, Uncle Charlie, the neighbor, the Internet or the government than we do in Almighty God.

No matter how much research you do running around trying to figure out what to do, you will never get a better deal anywhere than what Jesus won for us on the cross. Make it a habit to always consult Him first, trusting that when it comes to your well-being, He will always say "Yes!"

Stop Perishing!

If you ever memorized scripture as a child (if you didn't, start now!), one of the first verses you probably learned was John 3:16: "God so loved the world that He gave His only begotten son, that whosoever believes in Him will not perish but shall have everlasting life." I remember the day my little gold star went up on the board in Sunday School for that one!

I've been mulling over the word "perish", and asking God for enlightenment.

In an adult class at Sunday School recently we had a discussion about sickness and death. Did you know that some people think we have to have sickness so we'll die? The remark, "No we don't, we can just go home to be with the Lord," stimulated quite a discussion. We had to admit that we all knew people who just peacefully went to sleep and went home to be with the Lord with no trauma. We had to admit that scripture mentions lots of folks who went home to "sleep with their fathers." We had to admit that health is God's will and sickness is Satan's will, and we shouldn't mix the two plans in our own thinking.

As I keep pondering all this, I realize that some people are in the process of perishing all the time, moving from one illness or infirmity to another, fully expecting that one will eventually take them out. What's worse is they are convinced that this is God's plan.

If you have been one of that crowd, search the scriptures and ask the Holy Spirit to guide your understanding about this. Stop perishing today!

The Keys to Your Chariot of Fire

"For those who honor Me, I will honor..." (1 Samuel 2:30).

Honoring God in everything is critical to riding in victory in every aspect of life. Sickness and disease, oppression and stress, doubt and worry vanish into insignificance when we honor God with our faith, our attention, our trust, and our love.

One night, Moe and I watched his favorite film, *Chariots of Fire*,[5] which is a powerful real life story of the immeasurable power available to a man who honors God in all things. It squarely hits what we are up against: the factors that try to steal victory from us, and the simplicity of single-minded devotion to our Almighty God.

This movie is about real people in real time, and a real God who offers real victory. It shows us what we can and should be. Dishonoring God with sin, doubt, fear, distractions and everything else steals away the power and victory He so freely offers us. Honoring Him will get us out of the old, beat up rattletrap vehicle of our faith that we've been driving around and put us in the driver's seat of a vehicle beyond our wildest dreams: a chariot of fire! There are no speed limits on the road to victory!

Healing... On Easy Street

"For my yoke is easy, and my burden is light."(Matthew 11:30)

It is shocking how difficult it is for some people to receive and believe good news. Matthew Chapter 11 is worth reading from this perspective. John the Baptist sends two of his guys to check out Jesus' credentials. This is his cousin, whom Elizabeth recognized in Mary's womb.

Jesus replies by listing some of the healing miracles He has performed: the blind see, the lame walk, the dead are raised. Just how much evidence does a person need to get the message?

Yet even today, some believers have a struggle to believe that they can "just say NO" to any evil Satan has for them: sin, doubt, fear, sickness, disease, and adversity. Those of us who were blessed with godly, mature parents may have had the example that equipped us to say NO to temptation, so we avoided things like drug or alcohol abuse, theft, or sexual immorality that could have led to pregnancy out of wedlock, sexually transmitted diseases, or other consequences. Our parents and other people who influenced us may not have known we can also resist sickness and disease, so we grew up thinking that was an exception.

How sad to hear even believers say, "Oh, but sometimes you have to be realistic," meaning you have to set aside the glory to deal with suffering in the natural world. Yet Jesus promises that if we will come to HIM, He will give us rest. He urges us to take His yoke upon us and LEARN from Him, because He is meek and lowly of heart (his strength is disciplined; under control) and if we do we will find rest. Not, may I point out, so we can suffer with Him. His suffering is over, accomplished forever on the cross!

So when He invites us to take His yoke, it is not because He needs help with suffering. It is because, "My yoke is easy and my burden is light." We can receive and believe this when we know who Jesus really is, as John the Baptist and his guys had to know.

If your burden is not easy and light right now, ask Him to reveal Himself to you. He is waiting with open arms and great joy to welcome you to easy street!

Trust...Direction...Promise

2 Timothy 4:18: "The Lord will rescue me from every evil and save me for His heavenly kingdom. To Him be the glory for ever and ever. Amen."

Exodus 15:26: "If you will diligently hearken to the voice of the Lord your God, and do that which is right in His eyes, and give heed to His commandments and keep all His statutes, I will put none of the diseases upon you which I put upon the Egyptians; for I am the Lord, your healer."

Isaiah 55:12: "For you shall go out in joy, and be led forth in peace; the mountains and the hills before you shall break forth into singing, and all the trees of the field shall clap their hands."

Check with a Doctor

Recently a friend of ours who has a very powerful healing ministry sent a message concerning the importance of doctors. Does that surprise you? His point was this: if you have strongly developed your faith, you may be able to receive healing directly from God all the time, big or little healings; it makes no difference. However, if your faith is not yet developed, then at critical times the doctor can be your best friend.

Let's think about this. We do not need to pray for MORE faith, because scripture assures us that faith is a gift of the spirit and each of us has been given "the measure of faith" we will need for everything (Romans 12). However, we must exercise and strengthen that faith, and use it, obeying the guidelines of things we should do and things we should avoid to keep ourselves safe. Some of us spend a great deal of thought and time on doing everything popular current wisdom says we need to do to have fit, beautiful healthy bodies, but very little time searching for God's wisdom concerning the same.

Does your doctor want you well? God in His mercy uses doctors all the time to facilitate healing for those who are "not there yet" or are clueless about the power of faith, or even for those who are strong in faith and can provide a strong testimony for specific doctors or the medical community. We want to be sure that our doctors are walking in faith, too, and not leaning on their own scientific brilliance alone. Moe and I have two doctors: one is a general practitioner and the other practices holistic medicine. Both are delighted when they don't see us. They WANT us to be well! That's a pretty good asset for a doctor, wouldn't you say? Praise God for these wonderful men and women, and the nurses and others in the medical community, who devote their lives to the well-being of others every day.

I always say we should go back to primary sources, such as the book of Luke. Luke was a physician. He was also one of those detail-oriented people, and his gospel includes tons of details the others don't include, probably for those of us who need tons of detail in order to be satisfied. I love the book of Luke because of these details, and also because I love to know how a physician viewed and reported the healings of Jesus. I double dog dare you to read the whole book thinking about doctors and faith as you do so. You are in for a treat if you are hungry for truth, in detail!

So today my suggestion is to check in with Dr. Luke immediately.

You will find that he recommends the Specialist, Dr. Jesus, every time!

Put Up or Shut Up, According to His Word

"For with God nothing shall be impossible. And Mary said, Behold the handmaid of the Lord; be it unto me according to thy word." (Luke 1:37-38)

The angel Gabriel is busy in the book of Luke. He appears to two people with news of an unexpected baby. First, Zacharias, whose elderly wife, Elizabeth, would bear John the Baptist. Second, Mary, a virgin, who would bear Jesus.

In both cases, the birth would be very unusual, and would require faith and obedience. Zacharias initially responds to the announcement with doubt, so God SHUTS his MOUTH. Gabriel explains that this is because he is filled with doubt and does not believe Gabriel's words, which would be "fulfilled in their season."

Mary responds differently. She does not reject the announcement. She does not ask why; instead, she asks "How?" When this is explained, she responds, "Be it unto me according to your word."

The bottom line is that with God, nothing is impossible when we are willing to receive, believe, and act on His Word.

When we or a loved one are attacked by sickness, disease, or injury do we respond with faith and trust in God's word concerning His will for us in these things, or do we question in doubt? Is the response that comes out of our mouth obedient to His will?

If we have the trust of Mary, we will rejoice: "My soul doth magnify the Lord, and my spirit hath rejoiced in God my savior" (Luke 1:46-47 KJV). It will then be done to us according to His Word.

If our faith still needs exercise, we would be wise to shut our own mouths, as God shut the mouth of Zacharias, so that we do not contradict and counteract the Word and Will of God for our healing.

Current vernacular says: "Put up or shut up!" Whichever you choose, may it always be according to His Word.

First Fruits of Faith

When I was five my expectant mother and I were living with my godmother in California while my father was fighting in Korea. One day in church there was a teaching on tithing, which Mom and Aunt Susie discussed at great length over Sunday dinner. For a lesson on tithing go to Matthew and turn left to the last book of the Old Testament and read Malachi 3:8-10.

I was fascinated, and asked if I could tithe. Mom explained that I could do that only when I had worked to earn money, because the first fruits must come from our own labor. Think about that in light of our entitlement society. Imagine the blessings people miss if they neglect the power of the first fruits of their own labor. I woke up the next morning very early thinking about all this, and came up with a plan.

I got dressed, grabbed a pad of paper and a pencil, and began to ring doorbells up and down the street in the neighborhood. I told the bewildered people just having their breakfasts that I was selling cookies. Would they like to buy oatmeal or chocolate chip? My mom made both, and they were great! They asked me how much the cookies would cost, and I said I didn't know. Even so, I got tons of orders! I really couldn't write well yet. I just made marks on the pad. Finally, my frantic mother found me.

There's a lot here in this funny little story that can help us with our faith walk concerning healing. First, even as a little child I grasped the advantage of the tithe, and the idea that God very much wanted to bless us but we had to take some action too. I also understood, with Mom's coaching, that I had to personally take some responsibility. I marched out in total faith that people would give me money for those cookies, and wonder of wonders, adult people actually were ready to do that! Finally, I did not have any idea of what to say when they asked me the cost.

I do not know what it cost Jesus on the cross to pay the debt of my sin and suffering, my sickness and disease, my fear and lack. But the same innocent faith that I had back then assures me that the price was paid in full, and that if I will follow the Lord's loving prompting and work to tithe on my faith and my substance, increase will surely follow.

All of the bad things no longer belong to me because the full price was paid. Alleluia!

"Lord, may the first fruits of our faith yield the blessings of life and health you promise in Your Word, and may we keep our hearts with all diligence, knowing that out of them flow the issues of life. With heartfelt gratitude in Jesus' name we pray. Amen."

Christmas Every Day!

We are created by a God "...who wants all people to be saved and to come to a knowledge of the truth" (I Timothy 2:4).

He does not want us to suffer defeat and sorrow: "Do I take any pleasure in the death of the wicked? declares the Sovereign LORD. Rather, am I not pleased when they turn from their ways and live?" (Ezekiel 18:23)

"For God did not send His Son into the world to condemn the world, but to save the world through Him" (John 3:17).

"For the grace of God has appeared that offers salvation to all people" (Titus 2:11).

Do you get it? The fact is that God has an unchanging desire to provide good things for His beloved children. This should be clear to anyone who seriously studies scripture and asks the Lord for understanding. We do not have to earn these wonderful things. We do not have to bribe God or tip Him! It's not what WE do that has the power; it is what He has already done for us because He loves us!

We recently had a young guest in his early twenties speak for us at a business meeting, and one of the things he said was this, "Every one of us can be blessed, but you need to be blessable!" We can't earn the blessing because it is given freely, but we need to think and behave in such a way that we can receive the freely offered blessing.

In terms of health and healing, how does this apply? Have you, or anyone you know, tried to EARN health? Done all the right things current wisdom suggests? Doing that is not a bad idea, of course, but there is something both much simpler and deeper here. Are we "healable?"

Our heartfelt desire for the Lord, a desire that reaches out to Him daily, studying His word, spending time with Him in prayer "without ceasing" throughout the day and as we fall asleep at night, striving to keep His commandments and "walk in His ways," loving Him and loving His children (even the unlovable ones), and receiving His blessings rather than ignoring or rejecting them are all things that help us to become "blessable" and "healable!"

Little children who know they are loved can rush to their stockings on Christmas morning, knowing there will be wonderful surprises inside. Not scorpions, thorns, or rocks, but wonderful things! They have not earned these things—although they may have tried very hard to be good—these are gifts freely given by someone who loves them very much, and takes delight in their joy. It is the same for our Heavenly Father, who takes joy in us when we are blessable, healable, and willing to receive all the fullness of the love He has for us.

Batter Up!

"For God hath not given us the spirit of fear, but of power and of love and of a sound mind." (II Timothy 1:7)

"Is any among you sick? Let him call for the elders of the church, and let them pray over him, anointing him with oil in the name of the Lord, and the prayer of faith will save the sick man, and the Lord will raise him up; and if he has committed sins he will be forgiven. Therefore confess your sins to one another that you may be healed. The prayer of a righteous man has great power in its effects." (James 5:14-16)

Have you heard this before? Really? Have you heard and paid attention and obeyed? Do a little interview with yourself to find out!

1) When you seek healing are you fearful/timid/uncertain or powerful/trusting/certain?
2) How are you doing with the love part? Are you bitter, envious, angry, disdainful, or estranged regarding anyone?
3) Have the elders of your church prayed over you, anointed you with oil, prayed in the name of the Lord, in faith?
4) Have you confessed your sins "to one another" and been forgiven? It says those sins "will be forgiven."

James assures us that if these things are in place we are in position to be healed. Think about baseball: if you are the catcher and you are not behind the plate, there is no way you can do your job, no matter how many balls are pitched. If you are the pitcher and persist in pitching to the stands, there is no way the batter can be effective. We can't expect a home run if we are running around like batters who neglect to pick up the bat.

These are not hard directions, nor are they complicated. If they are to have "great power in their effects"...we have to do them.

Pass/Fail and Graduation

"You make known to me the path of life in your presence there is fullness of joy; at your right hand are pleasures forevermore." (Psalm 16:11)

"I call heaven and earth to witness against you today, that I have set before you life and death, blessing and curse. Therefore choose life, that you and your offspring may live" (Deuteronomy 30:19).

Do you really think that God would tempt and taunt us with something we could not have? Surely not! That is not the way our God deals with His beloved children! In the scriptures above, He is letting us know that fullness of joy, pleasures ever more, life and blessings are available to us and to our offspring.

Note, however, two things: 1) We must choose to receive these blessings, and 2) We will find them in His presence. Our health and wellness are clearly part of joy, pleasures forevermore, and choosing life!

I am remembering a student I had one year while teaching high school English. The goal was to empower students to effectively communicate by understanding what others are expressing and by making themselves understood by others through language. In one particular class, required for graduation, discussion participation was key and therefore a major part of the final grade. One of the seniors had completed all the written work, but refused to participate in the critical discussion in spite of many reminders.

As the year drew to an end, it became clear that she would not pass the course and therefore could not graduate. The reality of this hit her parents first, who then promptly discussed it with her. All three came to me to ask what could be done, so I outlined for her exactly what participation in discussion she needed to demonstrate in the final two weeks of school in order to pass the course.

The change in her was remarkable! You never saw such participation! She listened to the other students, responded with comments and questions, and offered ideas of her own. She became a great communicator. At graduation she came to me to tell me what a difference this experience had made for her. She truly had not realized that she was capable of this, nor how valuable it was to her. She made it a point to let me know that allowing her the choice to fail or to succeed had opened up the way to a very different future for her, and the ability to communicate would make a huge difference for her in her future life.

We too are fully capable of participating in the health and wellness God desires for us, and we don't have to wait until the eleventh hour to obtain it.

God allows us to choose: fullness of joy or just a little, pleasures forevermore or just now and then; even life or death. Be assured that IN His PRESENCE we can make the best choices!

How do we place ourselves in His presence? He tells us very simply:

"Draw near to God, and He will draw near to you. Cleanse your hands, you sinners, and purify your hearts, you double-minded." (James 4:8)

"And without faith it is impossible to please Him, for whoever would draw near to God must believe that He exists and that He rewards those who seek Him." (Hebrews 11:6).

Choose to participate today, pass the course, and celebrate an amazing graduation!

A Life Sentence

So shall my word be that goes forth from my mouth; it shall not return to me empty, but it shall accomplish that which I purpose, and prosper in the thing for which I sent it." (Isaiah 55:11)

God says what He means and means what He says. You may know some people who are like that, too. I do! However, God's word also accomplishes what He says. That's why it is so important for us to line up our words with God's words when it comes to healing.

1. The adventure begins when we realize that God is good, loves us, wants us well, and tells us how to get and stay that way.
2. It continues when we seek the scripture to find out exactly what He does say.
3. It comes to glory when we say what He says and do or avoid what He directs, and we get well!
4. We get the results He speaks, wills, and promises!

There are people who don't know the truth in that first step. Then there are people who know that much, but don't follow through as in the second step. There are people who do that, but fail to follow through with the action of the third step. But then there are the people who go all the way and live their lives in the fourth step.

Sometimes people mumble and grumble and whine and moan like life was a "life sentence." You live in the fourth step above and your grumbling days will be over! When your life is the life sentence GOD speaks for you, you are in for the adventure of a lifetime and beyond!

Psalm 91: The Insurance/Assurance Policy

"I will say of the Lord, He is my fortress, my God: in Him will I trust" (Psalm 91:2).

Psalm 91 is a great scripture to memorize and repeat daily. It has been called our "divine insurance policy." Read through it and ask yourself if you've ever been offered a more comprehensive policy any time, anywhere, for any amount of money!

Most of us have purchased insurance policies in our adult lives: auto insurance, health insurance, homeowners and even extra policies for jewelry or furs. Can you imagine paying on those policies for years only to fail to claim them when the disaster hits?

We purchase the policies anticipating that something awful may happen, then pay on them for years so we can feel prepared. Why would we not cash in on that should the anticipated circumstances come to pass?

Psalm 91 is insurance and assurance that we are covered. No matter what, God is our safety net! How do we stake our claim when the time comes? Hebrews 10:23 instructs us: "Let us hold fast the profession of our faith without wavering; for He is faithful that promised."

The temptation is to focus on the disaster rather than the insurance. Think about this. When you are believing for health but experiencing symptoms, what are you thinking about most? When someone asks, "I know you are believing in faith, but how are you feeling?" isn't there sometimes a longing to say how we feel and receive that comforting sympathy? Sadly, for some people the only love and caring they ever receive from others happens when they are ill, so illness itself becomes desirable in order to receive the longed-for sympathy which passes for love.

The fact is that sympathy feels good for a few minutes, but healing feels good for a long time! I have a friend who stepped on a big darning needle when she was in high school. It went deeply into her foot and was horribly painful. All her friends gathered around her and their caring and sympathy surrounded her. Then a girl she didn't even know well reached over and pulled out the needle! She still expressed the relief of that moment when she was telling me the story many years later!

Doesn't it just make sense to claim our insurance policy from God, get the needle out of our foot, and move on?

The Body, A Sacrifice of Worship

"I appeal to you therefore, brethren, by the mercies of God, to present your bodies as a living sacrifice, holy and acceptable to God, which is your spiritual worship"(Romans 12:1).

Do you ever wonder why out of all eternity God chose to give each of us a brief life in the flesh? What could be the reason for this fleeting time in a temporal, impermanent world out of all eternity, spiritual and endless? These are huge thoughts, too big for the human mind to fully comprehend. Our time in this state is so brief, but must be so very important. What do we need to learn here that we would not learn outside this life?

The scripture from Romans tells us that we can offer our bodies as a holy sacrifice to God, as spiritual worship. We can offer what is temporary, confined in the flesh, to the one who is permanent, unchanging, and vast. Clearly our desire should be to offer ourselves "pure and holy" to the Lord.

Where am I going with this? God has given such specific directions about how to keep ourselves pure and holy, but maybe we have read them with a motive of staying safe, forgetting that we can at the same time be offering these states as a sacrifice of worship.

When Solomon honored his father David's desire by finishing the temple, he worshipped God and then rose to bless the people. He asked that God would "Incline our hearts unto Him, to walk in all His ways, and to keep His commandments and His statutes, and His judgments which He commanded our fathers" (I Kings 8:58). Here we see wise Solomon's perception of right and holy living as a form of worship as well as a path to well-being.

Suddenly, I see that the well-being of my body can be a form of worship, when I offer it in all my choices, actions, and desires as a means of worship. Solomon goes on to note in verses 60-61: "That all the people of the earth may know that the Lord is God, and that there is no other. Let your heart therefore be perfect with the Lord, to walk in His statutes and to keep His commandments." We learn that worship through our physical flesh can be our testimony.

No wonder Satan is so determined to trip us up to defile our bodies with sin or inflict them with sickness and disease. We know that to walk in God's ways and lean on Him is the way to live in order to avoid that trap. Today I also see that offering our bodies as a living sacrifice in worship is another profoundly powerful way to experience His perfect will for us, spirit, soul and body.

Let's remember this as we worship in our churches. Remember the lessons of that temple built so long ago, where "the glory of the Lord filled the house of the Lord." (8:11) May we offer our own bodies as temples in which He will dwell forever.

Health Assessment!

I love the story in Acts 28 about Paul being bitten by a venomous snake. He and his team had just overcome shipwreck and were being helped by "a barbarous people" who showed them kindness and had built a fire to warm them. Paul was throwing some wood on the fire when the viper bit him, to the horror of the natives who knew the snake's deadly venom and expected immediate swelling of his arm followed by death. Paul, however, knew he was safe and simply shook the snake off with no ill effects. They were then taken to the home of a man names Publius, where Paul laid hands on his host's gravely ill father and healed him. (v. 8) Then other sick people were brought to him and were also healed.

How wonderful! How powerful! Here is Paul, simply obeying what Jesus said we should be able to do. Are we as prepared as Paul was? If not, why aren't we?

While in the middle of reading Acts, I received an email from a business friend requesting a document. It was a twenty question Health Assessment. If any of the twenty items is a health issue for someone, the suggested vitamin/mineral is indicated. Not being a believer in coincidence, I started thinking! Maybe we need to assess our own state of spirit, soul, and body to determine what we might need to do to strengthen our own ability to 1) fight off attacks on us and 2) strengthen our faith so that we too can lay hands on the sick for their healing.

I'm mulling over what my twenty questions need to be!

1) Have I stayed firmly in the Word on a daily basis?
2) Have I lined up my belief with what God says, not what other people say or what I feel?
3) Have I kept the Commandments?
4) Have my words been words of faith, and not fear or doubt?
5) Have I praised God continuously for His faithfulness in fulfilling His promises?
6) Have I shared the good news with others?

Make your own list, and assess yourself.

Venom is defeated through Christ Jesus, so watch out, snakes! Let's shake them off with Paul and get on to the work of healing God's beloved children as He has instructed His followers to do.

Nancy Drew Investigates

One day as I sat down with my Bible, God sent the word "establish" to my mind. Establish? How does that concept help us overcome sickness and disease? I figured I would check the concordance in the back of the Bible to see if that word was even listed. Wow! I thought there might be a couple of references, but there is a whole list. As I began to look them up, I realized that being established in the way of God's covenant and direction is very frequently stressed in the Word. I then went online to find the scriptures I might want to include in this message and there were pages and pages of references on the word establish.

Clearly this is something very important for us, so your clueless but fearless "healing message" girl is on to the investigation like Nancy Drew, Miss Marple, Agatha Christie, Dorothy Sayers, Sherlock Holmes, and Mycroft. Isn't this fun?

Let's start with Proverbs 4:20-27, which actually begins with a mention of health:

"My son, attend to my words; incline thine ear unto my sayings. Let them not depart from thine eyes; keep them in the midst of thine heart. For they are life unto those that find them, and health to all their flesh. Keep thy heart with all diligence; for out of it are the issues of life. Put away from thee a froward mouth, and perverse lips put far from thee. Let thine eyes look right on, and let thine eyelids look straight before thee. Ponder the path of thy feet, and let all thy ways be established. Turn not to the right hand nor to the left: remove thy foot from evil."

Clearly we are to ESTABLISH ourselves, our thoughts, words, and deeds, in the Almighty God, our creator and Heavenly Father, who has established a covenant with us. We are to obtain and maintain life and health by focusing without deviation on His ways with our minds and hearts (vs. 21, 23;26), our ears (20), our eyes (attention) and our mouths (24) without straying away.

Our Father knows His customers here. He knows that in this fallen world we will be distracted and tempted away from His way of safety. If you will go back to the beginning of Chapter 4, in the first two verses He speaks to each of us directly as a loving father:

"Hear, ye children, the instruction of a father, and attend to know understanding. For I give you good doctrine, forsake ye not my law."

And following the chapter, the first words in Chapter 5 are:

"My son, attend unto my wisdom, and bow thine ear to my understanding…"

My deep hope is that each one of us will take these passages for what they truly are: a personal message from our loving God who wills that we walk in health and safety all the days of our lives. It's as if Daddy was saying, "Here's an extra $20 just in case you need it. Here are the keys to the car and well, here, just use my credit card." Why? Because He loves you!

"Heavenly Father, thank you for loving us so much. Thank you for holding our hands as we cross the dangerous streets of life. Should we wander away sometimes like little children, thank you for being there with your arms of protection wide open to receive us once again. Help us to establish ourselves on the paths you have revealed to us. We receive your instruction today, and ask that you will give us the attention, strength, and wisdom to walk steadily and firmly in the path you have established for us until the end of that path brings us safely home to you forever. In Jesus name, Amen."

We're Number One!!!

A dear and respected friend commented recently, "If you want to receive blessings by the bushel you need to go to the Word with a bushel basket." Smack! Are we going to the Word and are we toting the biggest basket we can possibly take?

I'm reminded of Simon Peter when Jesus told him and his fishing buddies, who had just returned from a VERY unsuccessful day, to let down their nets one more time (Luke 5:4). Peter figured a carpenter probably didn't know more about fishing than a professional like himself, but he was polite enough to let down ONE net. Of course, the net was filled and the boat was filled. You know how God overdoes it when He wants to bless us, which is ALL the TIME, by the way!

Scripture tells us we don't receive because we don't ask, and that when we do, "The Lord is able to give you much more than this." (See II Chronicles 25:9). God's goodness is only limited by our capacity to receive it.

Are we hesitant to ask for, believe for, and receive really big and important stuff? Afraid we're not being humble? Nonsense! Did you ever see football fans go to a tough game, intently watch and judge every play, and then when their team wins they scream, "We're number one!" They have not done a darn thing to play or win that game, they just bought a ticket! However, they have no problem claiming "We're number one!" when the victory rolls in.

We didn't do a thing to earn the right to health and healing. Even the ticket was bought for us by Jesus when He paid the price on the cross. But we surely have the right to stand on the bleachers and scream, "We're number one!" because in Him we absolutely are.

You'd Better Shop Around!

A lot of people do a lot of shopping around before they decide what to buy or what decision to make about something important, and I suspect health and healing can be a part of this process. Why do we shop around? Are we looking for the best deal? The most convenient? Readily available? Least expensive? What exactly is the motive?

Moe and I went to Wegman's yesterday. The moment I enter this amazing store I get overwhelmed! There's too much going on for a sanguine to take it all in and stay focused. Having a shopping list helped steer me to the right areas (well kind of). I needed some help from staff and friendly fellow shoppers on occasion, but there were so many options, such as organic or not, inexpensive or more expensive, familiar and unfamiliar and so on.

Do you ever feel that way in your journey to receive healing and health? There are indeed so many options out there: what Granny said or did, what the doctor or nurse said, or what you heard on TV or read on the Internet. What is the latest from medical science? Have you ever been shopping around? What on earth (literally!) are you going to put in your cart for this life in the flesh?

Like the grocery adventure, are we looking for the best deal? Easiest? Cheapest? Most easily accessible? Even searching the Bible may seem like trying to find your way in a vast, scriptural Wegman's. Moe contends that any decision based solely on price will generally be a bad decision. This may be true for convenience as well.

In finding our way to the healing that was bought and paid for at a price we could never pay, we may receive some help from the Lord's staff and other friendly shoppers who are on the journey with us. Thank God for them! However, shopping, no matter what it's for, is always a very personal thing, so God has provided us with what we need: scriptures with a concordance and direct access to Him personally. Now there's customer service that is truly divine!

Buyers beware! There are lots of resources you can check out, but none will have the 100% satisfaction guarantee freely provided by our

Heavenly Father. So when you're tired of shopping around, go for the home delivery of the very best, personalized plan exactly for YOU and all your shopping needs! Then you can relax and enjoy health and long life with no limited time coupons with your satisfaction guaranteed!

Finding your Ebenezer

We've considered some thoughts about shopping, and I'm still "in the store" today. At one point in my life when I was learning some very important information that was new to me, my mentor told me about the "Grocery Store Analogy." He pointed out that when you go to grocery shop you don't just take one of everything they sell. Your cart couldn't hold it all for one thing, and then you don't like everything they sell. He suggested that I view what seemed to be an overwhelming amount of information and just select the "cans" I could use at that time.

I followed this encouraging advice, and found I could digest the information a bit at a time and then go back and pick up more. I discovered that the cans I skipped the first time around turned out to be the very ones I needed the most later. I just hadn't been ready for them. As the Lord puts it, "I fed you with milk, not solid food, for you were not ready for it" (I Corinthians 3:2).

Learning about healing can be like this. The scripture can seem like a vast grocery store. There is just so much! Yet, as we take what we can digest and keep going back for more, eventually we find exactly what we need to bring the power of truth home to our bodies and our lives.

What are we shopping for? Yesterday in church we sang "Come Thou Fount of Every Blessing,"[7] a powerful hymn that includes the line about raising your "Ebenezer." This refers to a stone (I Samuel 7:12) set up as a memorial and reminder of God's constant, never failing help, no matter how hopeless the situation appears to be. I suggest that we need to be ready to find an Ebenezer for ourselves and select it from the shelf. It may be a selection of scripture, or a spirit-filled word from a hymn, or maybe a word directly from the Lord.

Whatever it is, seek and ye shall find! Be willing to move your faith from milk to meat. Move from the baby food aisle and grow up into the powerful, healing faith we find at the Father's table.

By the way, here are the words to that hymn. I strongly recommend that you go on YouTube and find the version sung by a

Mormon youth choir. Hearing it provided six of the most powerful and meaningful moments of my life.

> Come, Thou Fount of every blessing,
> Tune my heart to sing Thy grace;
> Streams of mercy, never ceasing,
> Call for songs of loudest praise.
> Teach me some melodious sonnet,
> Sung by flaming tongues above.
> Praise the mount! I'm fixed upon it,
> Mount of Thy redeeming love.
>
> Here I raise my Ebenezer;
> Hither by Thy help I've come;
> And I hope, by Thy good pleasure,
> Safely to arrive at home.
> Prone to wander, Lord, I feel it,
> Prone to leave the God I love;
> Here's my heart, O take and seal it;
> Seal it for Thy courts above.
>
> Jesus sought me when a stranger,
> Wandering from the fold of God;
> He, to rescue me from danger,
> Interposed His precious blood.
> Prone to wander, Lord, I feel it,
> Prone to leave the God I love;
> Here's my heart, O take and seal it;
> Seal it for Thy courts above.

The Secret of the Only Children

One of the most wonderful things a person can discover about God's nature is that He loves every one of us! No matter who we are or what we have done, He loves us, and that love means wanting the very best for us in every single way. Out of the abundance of God's heart, we have it made!

The scripture assures us that He is no respecter of persons (Acts 10:34). God used all kinds of people, good, bad and indifferent, to complete His plans on the earth. There were sinners, prostitutes, thieves; even Saul, His enemy, became Paul, His evangelist. When Jesus chose His disciples and leaders in the early church, He chose fishermen, tent makers, and even a physician! When He healed, He healed the blind, deaf, dumb, lame, fever ridden, demon possessed, palsied, and even the dead!

So what makes you so unique that He would exclude you?

What nonsense! We act as if He selected some special group for His favor, when in reality He selected every one of us as if we were His only son or daughter. Yet we act sometimes as if this reality was a big secret. If it is, this is a secret that needs to be told and manifested as the prayer book says, "Not only in our lips, but in our lives."

There is a wonderful little song I learned in Sunday School and have loved ever since. As I was checking the lyrics for this message, I discovered that it was also a favorite song of Elvis, who recorded it:

> *It is no secret what God can do*
> *What He's done for others, He'll do for you*
> *With arms wide open, He'll pardon you*
> *It is no secret what God can do.*[8]

What a simple statement of a profound truth. God is no respecter of persons. He is a loving father to each of His "only children!"

Bambi...and You

This week, a baby fawn who had just gotten control of its little legs came racing through our back garden so fast we thought it was a fox. It ran in huge circles through all the connected, open gardens around us. It returned to its mother for a milk break, then it was off again. That fawn was filled with pure joy! Don't tell me deer can't smile. That mother was beaming from ear to ear right along with us!

Just watching that wondrous event was so powerful that we are still talking about it. Moe was impressed with the reality that this little creature had not a single worry or fear in the world. I felt in my bones that this was the experience God has prepared for every one of us, the way He wants us to feel, the plan He had for us in the beginning! Total joy and no worries! Running back for certain refreshment to Him when we get thirsty! Then again to rejoicing in life!

Why do we not feel that every day? Why is seeing it an extraordinary rather than an ordinary event in human lives? Easy. If you were to list down all the experiences and feelings we encounter in human life on earth, and then went back to mark each one "the will of God" or "the will of Satan" you would begin to see.

The absolute conviction of God's glorious, abundant will for all that is good and wonderful for us becomes a question mark too often. Luke, the physician, writes this: "If a son asks for bread from any father among you, will he give him a stone? Or if *he asks* for a fish, will he give him a serpent instead of a fish? Or if he asks for an egg, will he offer him a scorpion?" (Luke 11:11-12).

He is quoting Jesus, who has just taught His people the Lord's Prayer. Jesus promises, "For every one that asks receives; and he that seeks finds; and to him that knocks it shall be opened" (Luke 11:10).

He then marches out to deal with a demon! I'm not making this up, go read Luke chapter 11. It is quite an eye opener.

Any person, if asked whether God wants us to sin, would say "NO" with conviction, unless they have chosen the occult and Satan is their god. Ask them does God want them to be sick. There should be the same firm "NO," but usually there isn't.

Breaking Ignorant

For a business conference, Moe and I developed a lesson titled, "Breaking Broke," which is about getting out of debt and living a debt free lifestyle. In the preparation process, I began to think about this in terms of healing and came to the conclusion that breaking broke and breaking sickness and disease are remarkably similar in that what we really need to break is ignorance. We get stuck where we are in life so often because we don't know what we don't know!

We're not stupid and we don't want to live in pain, but we can be ignorant about what to do about it.

Science has identified a concept called "cause and effect." Every effect has a cause. This applies to everything until you get back to the original "uncaused cause," which is a term some people use in place of the word "God." In my Dad's day, the almost universal belief in God came under attack, was questioned, diluted, and slowly removed from common consensus. As a scientist, he found this astonishing, as did many of his friends in the scientific and medical communities. He pointed out to me that God was the Uncaused Cause, a term designed to identify who/what God was with the following properties: omnipotent (all powerful), omnipresent (everywhere), omniscient (all knowing), and benevolent (perfectly good).

He also pointed out, in a discussion of cause and effect, that this was no new scientific idea, but was clearly described in the Bible all the way from "In the beginning, God..." throughout. Scripture is full of conditional statements that are often blunt: if you do this, then that is going to happen. Guidelines are clearly given. The Ten Commandments are a perfect example of this.

George Washington Carver was a remarkable man who achieved remarkable things in both a scientific and a spiritual manner. If you have not read *The Man Who Talks with the Flowers*[9] it is worth the trip. He realized that the "secrets" of the material world are available to us if we'll just pay attention.

Scripture tells us this over and over! "Taste and see that the Lord is good" (Psalm 34:8) is just one example. Malachi 3:10 challenges us to tithe and then see that God will "...open up the doors and windows of heaven." It's all over scripture and everywhere in life. The poet Edna St. Vincent Millay exclaims, "God, I can push the grass apart and lay my finger on thy heart!"

It is clear to anyone who pays attention that there are answers to the pain and suffering we encounter in the world. Our enemy uses ignorance to our disadvantage, while wisdom "cries from the streets" (Proverbs 1:20), offering us an option away from the confusion of ignorance to the wisdom of God.

My scientific dad commented that we need to draw our attention from the evils of this world "as it is" if we want to overcome them, and focus on the world as God planned it to be. Only then can we "break broke" and "break sick." I think George Washington Carver would agree. Do you?

Lead Us Not into Temptation But Deliver Us from Evil…

When I was born, my mother started filling in a baby book for me, with stats, pictures, and the fun events of my first seven years. There are cute little rhymes. One page, titled "Health Record" contains this rhyme:

> "Sometimes I had to stay in bed
> While other children played instead
> But Mother was so kind, you see,
> She served delicious toast to me,
> Told me stories, read me rhymes,
> I liked to stay in bed sometimes."

Has it ever been to your advantage to be sick? Was that the time, or is it now, that other people paid attention to you, were nice to you, and served you? Was that the valid reason to stay home from school, or call in sick from work? Are others so dependent on you, or demanding of you, that the only way you get to rest is by being sick?

This has been the story for many people. It is the way illness entered their lives and over time became a stronghold. Please understand, I am not saying kindness to each other when we don't feel well is wrong. No indeed! That comfort is an expression of love we all need to both give and receive. However, we need to be vigilant to avoid being led into temptation.

The Lord's Prayer includes, "…and lead us not into temptation but deliver us from evil."

"Dear Father, help us to avoid the temptation of the 'advantages' of being sick leading us into temptation that opens the door for the evil to enter our lives and invade our flesh. Deliver us from that evil possibility, and grant us wisdom and discernment so that we are able to avoid rather than embrace illness, and enter instead into the kingdom and the power and the glory, forever! Amen."

How Do You Know if It's Real?

How many times have you been "in love?" How many puppy love crushes, wishful thinking, or plain lust did you have to go through in your search for the real thing? High school and college are notorious times for this, and immaturity or ungrounded behavior can cause a lot of pain and destruction as we wonder: "How do you know if it's real?"

Remember all the foolish arguments and justifications? "It's OK if you REALLY love the person" has caused more train wrecks in more lives than we can count. The strong desire for the "REAL thing" can tempt us to squander fulfillment through ungodly choices and behavior on the journey to seek and find it. Then disillusion can set in, opening the door to doubt and fear.

When it comes to healing and the other signs and wonders that follow the authentic action of God in our lives, the same process can happen. Recently someone we respect shared that he belonged to a church for a while where people simply pretended. There was a false show of behaviors that were assumed by people looking for the real thing. He became so disillusioned that he started to doubt the possibility of the reality. He became afraid to believe, and so he cut himself off in a protective shell, while limiting himself to trust in his own reason and scripture alone to see him through.

Scripture, of course, leads us smack back into reality! Scripture does not fearfully avoid signs and wonders, it celebrates them. The Gospel is a fearless message. "Fear" has sometimes been defined as "false evidence appearing real." False evidence may steal the truth from people, just as false religion can steal the trust and hope of a sincere believer.

No matter how many puppy love or shabby substitutions are out there, the real thing is wondrous and, well, REAL! When we fall in love with the Source of all love, the signs and wonders fulfill us in every way that our hearts most deeply desire, and we can embrace all the joy God intended for us in a happy, healthy, fearless reality in this life and the next. The best news is this: <u>He is already in love with us</u>.

"Behold what manner of love the Father has bestowed on us, that we should be called children of God!" (I John 3:1).

On Earth as it Is in Heaven!

When we pray the Lord's Prayer, we pray "… thy will be done on earth as it is in heaven." Don't we? This comes from the lips of Jesus, so we certainly need have no argument or confusion about it being right to pray for this. Do you think there is sickness and disease, or any evil thing in heaven? NO! Here we see that we have the right to ask for the same here on earth, because that's what Jesus Himself prayed.

Do you think Jesus would teach people to pray something that was wrong or impossible? Of course not!

I am emphasizing this because so many people are afraid to believe the perfect will of God and to ask for it and to receive it right here, right now. They have a twisted sense that God is behind evil as well as the good things that happen. News flash: God is not a God of destruction! He is a God of healing and wholeness.

Let's look at Elijah's experience of this. "Then He said, 'Go out, and stand on the mountain before the Lord.' And behold, the Lord passed by, and a great and strong wind tore into the mountains and broke the rocks in pieces before the Lord, but the Lord was not in the wind; and after the wind an earthquake, but the Lord was not in the earthquake; and after the earthquake a fire, but the Lord was not in the fire; and after the fire a still small voice."

So it was, when Elijah heard it, that he wrapped his face in his mantle and went out and stood in the entrance of the cave. Suddenly a voice came to Him, and said, "What are you doing here, Elijah?" (I Kings 19:11-13).

There were times when God was in strong wind (on the Day of Pentecost when the Holy Spirit fell), and in an earthquake (when Paul and his friends were released from prison) and fire (when the Hebrew children were in the fiery furnace but did not burn, and the burning bush Moses encountered), but in all these cases, wonderful things, not destructive things, happened.

God is always with us in every experience: "I will never leave you nor forsake you" (Hebrews 13:5) but that does not mean the experience itself was His will, not if it is destructive, not if it is not "as it is in heaven."

This understanding should set us free to request and to receive God's perfect will, and refuse to be shackled by the evils we may encounter in this life. Let's mean it when we pray for things "on earth as they are in heaven..." and see what happens!

And I Don't Mean "Maybe!"

Our God is not a God of "maybe." Remember when your mom or someone else in your childhood had the authority to say, "Yes, no or maybe," to your ardent requests? Remember times when you used to hang on the answer? You had the request, but she had the power.

It's a funny word—and state of mind. Will it happen or not? It may be true or not.

Can you imagine scripture, and all life, if God were a maybe God?

God said, "Let there be light" and maybe there wasn't? God said if we confessed with our lips and believed in our hearts we could receive salvation, or maybe not. His way is the truth and the light, sometimes? He is always faithful and will never leave us or forsake us, possibly?

Someone gave me one of those little wooden frames with the words, "Faith is not just knowing God can, it's knowing that He will."

Looking at it squarely in the face, God seems to be a straight up yes or no kind of God. He does give us some conditional statements, however. "If you do ____, then ____will happen." On the whole, however, scripture is not that ambiguous!

The point? When we go to Him in prayer our expectation needs to be that what He says is exactly what He will do. My mom and dad used to say, "And I don't mean maybe!" when they were being absolutely firm! Ever hear that?

I think that's God. When He promises something He doesn't mean maybe. If we expect anything less than His promises we should not be surprised if we get results less than His promises.

I'm going to offer you a suggestion here. I think we should only ask God for things we know are His will for us, as revealed by scripture, not as revealed by well-meaning but vacillating friends, family, or sometimes even clergy. I think we should not bother praying over "maybes" that are full of human doubt. The God who loves us answers prayers of faith every single time. Remember He changes not!

We can count on Him and trust Him for His very best, yesterday, today, and forever. And I don't mean maybe.

Denying Jesus

It is probably an impossible idea to you that you would ever deny Jesus, under any circumstance. I surely have felt that too, but today the Lord lead me to Acts 3 for some new insights.

This contains the story of the man born lame. All of his life he had been carried to a gate outside the temple to beg for money. One day when Peter and John were about to enter the temple, the man asked them for money. They stopped and looked at Him, and Peter said, "Look on us" (3:4), so he did, expecting to receive money from them. Instead, they gave him an instruction: "In the name of Jesus Christ of Nazareth rise up and walk" (3:6). Well of course, he went ballistic, dancing and leaping into the temple with them to praise God. Wouldn't you? Or would you?

The scripture tells us that all the people who knew this man well were filled with wonder and amazement, but not faith. They made a big deal over Peter and John, who set them straight saying, "Why do you look so earnestly at us, as though by our own power or holiness we made this man to walk?" (3:12). They confronted the people with the fact that they had rejected Jesus, but "through faith in His name" (3:16) the lame man was now perfectly sound, right in front of their eyes.

How often do people who are sick or injured depend on other people for help, looking for "alms" in a contemporary way? This may be help from other people to carry us to the "gate", or to give us money, or whatever. Friends and family may behave the way the blind man's folks did, helping all they can. All the time, Jesus stands quietly, waiting for faith in HIM.

We may believe that Jesus is the Son of God who died for us and won us our salvation. We may believe that we will one day live with Him forever in heaven. But do we believe that He will heal us? Or do we deny that His compassion and power are still in effect?

Is it possible that we are denying His power, or His love for us, and in that way denying Him?

"Lord Jesus, we come to You like the lame man now freed from his disability for all these centuries. We come to You with his expectation and his faith. Please remove the scales from our eyes and the misunderstanding from our minds and the doubt from our hearts. Help us to know You as You truly are, not what others have said about You, but what You say to each one of us in a personal way today. We want to be dancing and leaping and praising You! We want everyone around us to know the wonderful power of Your love. May we never deny You in thought, word, or deed, instead let us be a shining light of faith and victory, giving you the glory as we receive the healing you long so deeply to give. In Your holy Name we pray, believing, Amen."

The Evidence: YOU!

The best evidence of God's unfailing love for His children, and for the Christian way of life in the power of scripture and personal relationship with Him, is US.

Consider this: our lives *should* be different from the lives of the pagans, or the worshippers of other gods, shouldn't they? What kind of evidence are WE as others are watching?

Matthew 4:23 tells us that manifestations are the proof or confirmation of the Gospel: "And Jesus went about all Galilee, teaching in their synagogues, preaching the gospel of the kingdom, and healing all kinds of sickness and all kinds of disease among the people." He taught about the good news, and then He went out and proved it!

Mark 16:15 and 20 tell us we should do what Jesus did: go into the entire world and preach the gospel to every creature.

"And they went out and preached everywhere, the Lord working with them and confirming the word through the accompanying signs."

John 14:12 gets even more pointed: "Most assuredly, I say to you, He who believes in Me, the works that I do he will do also; and greater works than these he will do, because I go to My Father."

Mark 16:20 tells us what happens to people who take God at His word and do what He directs: "And they went out and preached everywhere, the Lord working with them and confirming the word through the accompanying signs." Amen.

Any questions?

Sherlock...and You!

Christians should not be wandering around wondering what awful thing may happen to them next, in a state of fearful expectation. Christians should KNOW stuff. With all the 411 in scripture and 911 instantly available through the indwelling of the Holy Spirit, what on earth is all the drama about?

We don't need to be floating around in a murky pool of "what if this and what if that." We need to be sailing forward on a ship that never sinks because Jesus is on board, and we're with Him!

Both Matthew and Mark tell us the story of Jesus asleep on the boat when a storm comes up. The disciples start the fear drama and finally wake Him up. He immediately rebukes the storm, and then asks them "What is your PROBLEM?" Oops, I mean, "Why are you fearful? Where is your faith?" (Matt.8:23-24; Mark 4:38).

The way we carry on some days, He probably wants to ask us the same question.

Ignorance is no excuse, so acting like heathens and claiming, "I just don't know," will not cut it. Check out "knowledge" and "wisdom" in your concordance and get cracking. We have all the information we need, and more. Start investigating if this is a mystery for you.

People will spend hours, days, weeks or months searching for a car, a piece of furniture, a wedding gown, even a movie, but not ten minutes a day on vital information in the scriptures that is readily available and will save their lives.

It need not be that way. If you've fallen into that, slap yourself! Get cracking on solving that "mystery" that isn't a mystery at all. Jesus is alive and well on the boat, and ready to guarantee you a life of conviction. No more wandering and wondering! We KNOW the truth and the truth will set us free to go out and wonder instead about what will be the next marvelous, glorious, exciting adventure God has in store for us in this world and the next.

Chastening for the Clueless

As a clueless child, I needed the instruction and correction of my parents to survive. Didn't you? Sometimes they had to chastise me because I was heading into danger as fast as my little feet would take me!

Can you imagine such a parent saying, "I'll get out of the car and drive over her a couple of times to teach her not to run out into the street," or "I'll hold her hand on the hot stove burner to teach her to keep away from it." It is horrifying to think of a parent "disciplining" a child in such a way. A friend who worked with abused children in a local hospital once told me of the terrible story of a baby whose parent made him sit in a frying pan on the stove until his bottom was burned every time he soiled his pants, as toilet training.

We cannot imagine such cruelty, and certainly not as a way to teach lessons. Yet people accuse God all the time of inflicting or allowing sickness, disease, or injury to "teach us something." What hideous defamation of character! What heresy!

I needed to correct my own ideas about sickness versus healing, but God provided this teaching as a loving, compassionate father. He has corrected my wrong ideas by instruction, not cruelty:

"And you have forgotten the exhortation which speaks to you as to sons: My son, do not despise the chastening of the Lord, Nor be discouraged when you are rebuked by Him; For whom the Lord loves He chastens, And scourges every son whom He receives." (Proverbs 3:11)

"If you endure chastening, God deals with you as with sons; for what son is there whom a father does not chasten? But if you are without chastening, of which all have become partakers, then you are bastards and not sons" (Hebrews 12:5-8).

The word "chasten" means to correct by instruction. If we will receive that correction, repent of wrong thinking or actions or choices, we can literally save our lives.

"Now I rejoice, not that you were made sorry, but that your sorrow led to repentance. For you were made sorry in a godly manner, that you might suffer loss from us in nothing. For godly sorrow produces repentance leading to salvation, not to be regretted; but the sorrow of the world produces death" (II Cor. 7:9-10).

Of course, when we are in our clueless or suffering state God is right there with us, and indeed He will teach us. He will teach us, not BY suffering, but IN it when outside circumstances or we ourselves have brought it upon us.

We must choose to be open to instruction. Little children, and grown up little children, need to learn to seek chastening and instruction from their loving Father, through His Word and His indwelling presence. We need to pay attention to His warnings and His promises so that we will know how to "choose life."

"I call heaven and earth as witnesses today against you, that I have set before you life and death, blessing and cursing; therefore choose life, that both you and your descendants may live" (Deut. 30:18-20).

No Abracadabra

Have you ever been tricked? Have you ever been impressed by a magic act? Have you ever clung to a superstitious act sheepishly, or been amazed that other people believe in that stuff?

If so, it may explain why some people don't receive healing. They don't believe in it because they place healing in the same category as magic and superstition. For the same reason, people have left the church and the faith.

Healing is not a magic trick, a superstitious activity, or a roll of the dice. It is a matter of reverent faith, and needs to be approached with even more than the careful attention and persistence so many of us offer up when we work out, lose weight, win a game, or qualify for a degree.

Sometimes people, hearing the gospel for the first time, will receive Jesus, be filled with the Holy Spirit, and immediately receive healing. Sometimes this happens in very dramatic ways. God's grace is available to us all, but they are able to receive it immediately because they are in a state of having encountered truth without any interference.

Others, however, who have heard the gospel, been raised in a Christian home and gone to church their whole lives, still see healing as a form of a trick, which might work or might not. They may politely hold still for a minute to let someone pray for them, in a posture of "the flesh is willing but the spirit is weak."

These are people who have a, "Well, sometimes it works; sometimes it doesn't" attitude. They have not taken the time they need to seriously explore the possibility that scripture is true, and they may eventually fall away from the church, becoming "holly-lily" Christians, failing to pray daily; ceasing to pray before meals. The result of all this begins to prove to them that the faith is not valid, and this is convincing because their "faith" is not.

Calling on Jesus the Healer in faith is very different from shouting "abracadabra" or "open sesame" or even rubbing a rabbit's foot. It is also different from falling for the latest drug or treatment that is being advertised on television or in a magazine.

A clueless Christian can block your prayer with their flat unbelief, impatience, spiritual laziness, or thinly-veiled patronizing acquiescence to letting you pray for him. This kind of prayer will not be effective unless God intervenes with the same kind of thunderbolt Saul experienced when He became Paul.

Pretend religion and pretend faith can actually be superstitions. The most terrible thing about them is not just that they don't work, it's that they keep people from getting to the true religion and true faith which is real and powerful and effective. If your best defense is on the level of avoidance of black cats or walking under ladders, you are in trouble and so is anyone depending on you.

Finding the truth and walking in it takes effort, belief, and commitment without compromise. Don't wait for a stronger believer to pull rabbits out of a hat for you. Jesus our healer did not deal in magic tricks, and neither should we. People are not fed and satisfied with illusions. Those loaves and fishes were for real.

No Laughing Matter?

Anyone who knows me personally knows that I LOVE to laugh! I can see the funny side of almost anything going on, and have found that if you can do that you have a huge edge in overcoming the difficulties of life. Real laughter can snap things into perspective in a heartbeat. The scripture tells us that laughter is medicine.

"A merry heart does good, like medicine, but a broken spirit dries the bones" (Proverbs 17:22).

"A merry heart makes a cheerful countenance, but by sorrow of the heart the spirit is broken" (Proverbs 15:13).

"All the days of the afflicted are evil, but he who is of a merry heart has a continual feast" (Proverbs 15:15).

There are times, however, when we need to get serious. One example is when someone is facing serious illness.

In 2 Chronicles, when Solomon had completed the temple and was dedicating it, he called all the people together, and they began with tremendous praise, which is followed by the building being "filled with the presence of God and His Glory." Praise is serious and powerful. Then with everyone kneeling, Solomon reviewed their covenant with God, and requests "Let your word be verified" (6:17-18), "will you indeed dwell with men on the earth?"

God accepted the praise, prayer, and sacrifice of these people (7:1), and they concluded, "He is good: for His mercy endures forever" (7:3).

When we get serious before God, putting Him and His promises and His mercy FIRST, we can laugh at anything that comes against us. But we have to get serious first. We need to do this immediately when our health, safety, and well-being are first threatened or undermined in the little ways. We need to do it BEFORE bad things happen, and WHEN bad things happen. We can fully expect that His Word will be verified, because He does dwell with men in the earth, and His mercy does endure forever.

When we throw all that in the teeth of any affliction, it must bow its evil, defeated knee and flee before us. Let the laughter begin!

One of the funniest stories I know is about a man named Smith Wigglesworth, a man of such strong faith that he never took any guff from the enemy. One night he woke up from a sound sleep to see Satan sitting at the foot of his bed. He said, "Oh, it's only you," turned over, and went back to sleep.

Now THAT's a laughing matter!

Great News! Cool Water!

"As cold waters to a thirsty soul, so is good news from a far country" (Prov. 25:25).

We are experiencing what my kinfolk would have called "right smart heat" these past few days, and as a result I'm feeling really thirsty. When that's the case, nothing satisfies quite so well as plain old cold water. What a joy a glass of cold water is when you've been thirsty for a long time.

People are thirsty out there for the Good News of the gospel, especially in the area of healing. Have you ever watched people when someone is sharing a story about healing? Their faces are so transparent. Maybe there is reservation, doubt, or skepticism, but underneath there is eager, tentative hope. They WANT it to be true! The truth has a way of drawing us no matter how messed up our minds may be.

So today, I have a challenge assignment. Tell someone a story, a TRUE story, about healing. I LOVE it when I get these stories from you, and from other people. I love hearing them and I love telling them and I long to pass them on and on until the earth is buzzing with the joy of the good news of God's love and healing power.

Who will you tell? What story will it be? You may find that the person you told your story to will tell you their story in return. Keep swapping! You will find that this well never runs dry, and when one person's faith is strengthened in the telling, He will feel a deep desire to pass the stories on. Soon we are pouring out not just glasses of water, but pitchers of water and pools of water, and wells, and rivers and oceans!

I'll get you started. My friend Mark told me about God's healing power just in time for me to receive the healing of a tumor on my own brain. Now I specialize in praying out brain tumors! There have been several in our church families, and I've asked for specifics and then gone into prayer. I remind the enemy that he was defeated in MY head, and he's defeated in these heads too! Quietly, hesitantly, people are sharing that, "Well, the tumor has stopped growing and appears to be shrinking," and for some, the tumors are gone! I am not hesitant!

I KNOW that what God has done for me He will do for others. However, I always remember Mark, and the power of the testimony he shared with me when I really needed it.

So, who will you tell? And what story will you tell? Get out there and throw some cold water on Satan's plans today!

"I Do It!"

Little kids seem to go through a stage when suddenly they want to do things for themselves. They want to do everything from cutting their meat to stirring chocolate into their milk, trying to tie their shoes, to driving the car. Their constant demand is, "I do it! **I do it!**"

Let me ask you an honest, pointed question: do you want to be like Jesus? Do you sing about the longing for "a closer walk with thee?" "I want to be like Jesus" and other songs like that?

Have you noticed how many times we read in the scriptures, "Come unto me" and "fear not?" Do you skip over the bits where He tells us we should be doing what He is doing, and even greater things? What would all that mean if we took Him at His word and just grew to be more like Him?

For one thing, we'd be exclaiming, "I do it! **I do it!**" Then we'd be doing it.

Here's my picture. I see us having as many colds and headaches and tumors and illnesses as Jesus had. Now let's count them up. Uh, that comes to **ZERO!** I see us walking in health and victory, and healing people along the way just like He did. I see us cutting out the whining and wringing of hands over the illness that tries to come against us and others, knowing that it can be defeated because we saw Jesus do it, and we can do it too.

Some people think that it is prideful or blasphemous to try to think or speak or act like Jesus. Yet we know that this was the reason He took on flesh to walk with us in a body on this earth. Salvation, yes, but also to show us a perfect picture of how we are to conduct ourselves. He is the perfect example of what we are to do. Big tip: He TELLS US TO DO IT! I consider it more blasphemous not to obey Him and to snivel around like defeated orphans instead of children of God. Selah.

I see us as confident and excited as any little one attempting and succeeding in doing things for the first time and then mastering them!

Did you learn to swim, roller skate, ride a bike and/or drive a car? Got the picture?

How long has it been since you've had that glorious "I do it" feeling? What are you waiting for? Let me promise you, skydiving is nothing—a comparably boring event—compared to laying your hands in total faith on someone and feeling the power of God move through you with His healing touch.

Come on—adventure lies ahead! What will life be like when we are running around every single day living the "I do it" life God has planned for us?

Narrow the Choices to Two

We had a dear friend, recently deceased, who was a very successful businessman in great demand as a speaker. He was strong on the subject of business ethics, and even stronger on the conviction that business and personal ethics were linked. I can remember him saying, "It all boils down to God vs. Satan!" Because he spoke to mixed business crowds, he would add, "Or good vs. evil if that works for you; for a Christian they are the same thing."

When speaking to Christian audiences, such as when he was addressing a Sunday morning worship service, he would get more specific, backing his position with numerous scriptures from the Bible.

It came to mind this morning as I was mulling over the spirit/soul/body reality of our identities that this can apply to the battles of the flesh. We probably are aware of God vs. Satan when it comes to sins of the flesh. We are clear about which actions are the will of one and which are the will of the other!

When it comes to health and healing, are we as aware? Is it crystal clear to us that God wants us well and Satan wants us sick? Scripture is clear about God's will for His children, desiring all good things in abundance for us, and giving us guidelines and promises and grace and angels and all kinds of help for a great life while in the flesh on earth, even though man's control of the earth was lost at the fall.

The simple question, "Does God want this for me, or does Satan?" can clarify what is tempting, blessing, or attacking us at any moment. When making choices, asking, "Does this line up with God's will or Satan's?" is enlightening, to say the least.

Sadly, many people get conned into making a third choice based on their own, or another person's wisdom. This is a highly dicey proposition! It is adopted by people who don't believe in God and Satan or feel that they can make their own decisions in spite of the reality of these two forces.

It is also, even more sadly, adopted by many believers who forget whose they are, and neglect to dwell in the safety of God's will and protection.

Free will leaves our choices squarely in our laps. We will not consciously choose Satan's will for our sickness, injury, disease, but will we go directly to the will of our loving God, without a detour into our own wisdom.

The choice is ours. It seems clear to me that keeping our focus on God yields powerful and real and effective results to His glory and our well-being.

Rescue the Top for Your Toothpaste!

We surely recognize the importance of going to God first to find out what we are to do in a health situation. We know this is the best line of defense, but sometimes fear runs interference and we forget that. We know who the author of fear is, don't we? Hint: It ain't God.

Practicing the habit of going to God first in everything is a great way, and a practical way, to strengthen our faith muscle for the big deals. I want to share two personal examples.

1) Last night I took the plug out of my bathroom sink so the water would drain out more quickly. As I was waiting, I picked up my toothbrush and toothpaste, and the top of the toothpaste fell smack into the drain, bottom side up! It was too far down to reach, and I could not find any implement that would work in easing it out, remembering that if I turned it the wrong way it would fall farther into the pipe which would create greater plumbing adventures.

    I woke up and asked God what to do. Immediately, the thought came to put toothpaste on the end of the handle of my toothbrush. Made no sense to me, but I obeyed! The next thought was to gently lower the handle down into the top. I did, the top stuck to the toothpaste, and I raised both up. Victory!

God helps with dumb stuff like that all the time if we'll ask Him. He is never too busy or impatient!

2) A couple of nights ago, as I was washing my face, I happened to look under my jawbone on the left side to wipe away some cleanser and there was a round growth about the size of a dime. It was dark and plump. It was not a tick! It was more like a mole that had popped up suddenly. I tried rubbing it to see if it was just dirt,

but no, it was in my flesh. Feeling uneasy, I asked God what to do. Instantly, it was like I heard a chuckle and the thought came, "If the blood of Jesus can wipe away the sins of mankind, don't you think it can handle this mole?"

Well, I got the message, and wiped the thing and went to bed. Next morning I was washing my face and remembered the mole, which was now completely gone. I mean gone, completely vanished! Glory! What joy it is to wash and dry my face and praise God for it!

The key for me in all this is the chuckle. If we can grow close to God, close enough to feel His love, close enough to hear Him laugh, we can trust Him with all things, great and small because it's ALL SMALL TO HIM! How He chuckles when we turn to Him, so ready to help us in all things. How He must weep when we don't, and as a result go through such fear and pain.

Be encouraged to go to Him and listen carefully for that wonderful chuckle. Then you can put the top back on your toothpaste every single time! After all, if God is laughing, what do we have to worry about?

Do I Get it?

Do you remember when you first learned to ride a bike, or swim, or make piecrust? The first attempts were a little rocky, because you didn't quite get it. But then in one magic moment the bike glided off with you on it. Instead of sinking, you floated; the piecrust was light and fluffy and crispy and perfect.

Following trial and error, there is always evidence of success. If success is lacking, it does not mean that you can't do it, it just means that you don't get it yet.

Coaching by those who DO get it is important. Without those coaches we might try and fail for a long time, or never succeed. Their gift, and your perseverance, will finally pay off and you will do it. You get it! Following the coaching and the trial and error, the evidence—the fruit of success—is there for all to see and rejoice!

So how's your healing doing? Do you get it?

Healing is a GIFT from your coach the Holy Spirit. This, and the other Gifts of the Spirit can be found in I Corinthians 12. The Fruits of the Spirit are in Galatians 5:22-23. Two other gifts tend to accompany it: faith and miracles. More gifts kick in too, but let's keep it simple for now.

The evidence that you GET IT with healing is not only that you get healed, but that you expect healing in a very matter of fact way. Don't you LOVE that phrase? "MATTER of FACT!"

Someone commented recently to a group of us that when he came across someone in need of healing, he sent them to Moe because Moe had FAITH. Yes he does, but so do every one of us! God did not pick him out exclusively for that gift. The difference is, will we receive it? Will we exercise it?

There are many reasons why people don't get it. The primary reason is that Satan does not want us to get it. People don't know, and need a couple of those other gifts to help them out.

Another key reason is that, sadly, many people fear the Holy Spirit. It is hard to embrace what you fear, to let Him balance the bike for you, hold you up till you float, or show you how to knead the dough.

Getting to know this wonderful aspect of God and His love for us is so glorious and amazing! It changes everything when He is your comforter and teacher and guide and friend. When you trust Him and learn from Him, you'll be able to do so much: ride a bike, swim, make pie crust, get healed and so much more!

Do you get it?

Memory Work

Did you memorize things when you were a kid? I guess for school most of us did. I still have vivid memories of the times table and the Periodic table, but I mean things to inspire you. Did you memorize scripture or poetry?

As I was praying over this message, two examples from my past came to mind. Neither of which is in scripture, but both express ideas from scripture. The first was a poem given to me by my godmother to learn:

DID is a word of achievement,
WON'T is a word of retreat;
MIGHT is a word with a question,
CAN'T is a word of defeat.
OUGHT is a word of duty,
TRY is a word for each hour.
WILL is a word of beauty;
CAN is a word of power.

I didn't have to look this up because it has been with me since the day I memorized it.

The second was my framed quotation: "Faith is not just believing God CAN; it is knowing that He WILL."

As we consider our struggles in and growth through health challenges and healing victories, both of these take on rich meaning.

WON'T, for example, is a both a positive and a negative word. How defeating when we won't trust God, but how powerful when we WON'T give in or give up! How protective when we determine the things we WON'T do or think or speak because they can destroy us.

When TRY turns into CAN and CAN turns into DID, victories await us!

The second little quotation is brief but powerful. It expresses the contrast between those who believe God CAN heal and those who know He WILL. What a huge difference.

I suggest that all of us arm ourselves with additions to our memory banks that will have far more impact us then the times tables, the Periodic Table, or the Kings of England.

Memorize passages like, "By His stripes I am healed," "No weapon formed against me shall prosper," and "He who dwells in the secret place of the most high shall abide in the shadow of the Almighty!"

Made to Be Whole

In checking to see how long Adam lived on the earth (930 years), I read again about life before the fall, which was life as God planned it, and life after the fall. I noted the long lives of so many of our earliest ancestors, even after the fall.

The strong message I get every time I think about this is the contrast between the way God intended us to live, and the way we do live. Then I marvel over the fact that Jesus restored our ability to live as God wants us to on earth.

God didn't make us to be sick. In the Garden, there was no disease or injury; no discord or stress or sin; no wars or altercations or misunderstandings between men. There was no heavy workload. No pain, in childbirth or in anything else.

Instead, there was peace and joy and abundance. Try counting the leaves on a tree, the grains of sand on the beach, the number of bees buzzing around a hive or the ants running in and out of an ant hill or even the number of apples on an apple tree. Our God blessed us with heath and abundance out of His love! He had a glorious life planned for us, pain free.

Let the truth of that sink in. That's the way we are meant to live. What happened? We do not need to stand astonished in dewy-eyed innocence asking such a question. We know darn well what happened. The results of choosing ways contrary to the will and plan of God affected not only the person making that choice, but everyone else as well. Still happening, isn't it?

Just as the initial bad choice brought pain into the world, good choices can change things! Jesus brought a picture of the power of that change and then sent the Holy Spirit to dwell in us and put the power behind good decisions.

We have the right to rebuke and refuse all things contrary to the will of God. We can walk in that right, beginning the moment we give ourselves 100% to Jesus, turning our whole being and life—spirit, soul and body—over to Him, trusting His word, His work and His example to show us how to walk in victory.

No, we were not created to be broken. We were created to be whole.

Thinking about Your Thinking

If we take a moment to think about what we're thinking, it explains a lot! It has been said that fear and worry reflect greater faith in the problems from the enemy than faith in the answers from God. The kind of thinking that stews over the problems we face and tears us apart because we're trying to solve them by our own effort or that of other people can rob us of the belief necessary to receive the answer and walk in victory.

Moe was listening to a message this morning that focused on the ways unbelief can derail belief. Consider this:

"What if some did not believe? Shall their unbelief make the faith of God without effect?" (Romans 3:3)

"...I obtained mercy because I did it ignorantly in unbelief" (I Timothy 1:13).

"Take heed brethren lest there be any of you with an evil heart of unbelief, in departing from the living God" (Hebrews 3:12).

We can be distracted by unbelief through ignorance or through depending upon our own or other human "wisdom" rather than the promises of God.

I KNOW that other people and science and medicine have made vast advances, many of which were prompted by God's revelations. Alleluia! However, God's wisdom trumps them all, 100% of the time.

Jesus healed people left and right. We have encountered many scriptures describing how He "healed them all."

In Mark 6:4-5 we read that Jesus was unable to heal the people in His own hometown, except for a few, because of their unbelief!

What's the point? There are two:

1) Worry and fear are indicators that unbelief is performing an "interruption" in our faith.
2) We are paying more attention to the problems of man than to the promises of God.

Check yourself. Next time you worry or feel fearful, pay attention to what you are thinking about. If you're worried about how to solve a problem, or how to protect yourself or your family, then bingo! You are NOT thinking about the promises of God, the power of the blood of Jesus and His Holy Name.

Of COURSE, we can't solve our own problems. Of COURSE, He can!

Need help? It's there too. "And straightway the father of the child cried out, and said with tears, "Lord, I believe; help thou mine unbelief." (Mark 9:24). Guess what happened? The Lord did! The father's belief became stronger than his unbelief, and his son was healed.

So, here's a suggestion. The next time worry starts to creep in, ask yourself, "WHAT am I THINKING?" Immediately switch to God's promises, and rejoice! What He did for that father he'll do for you!

Right Now

One morning I flipped open my Bible and it opened to the first chapter of Mark, where I had written the words, "This is for right now!" in the margin. The verse next to that read, "The time is fulfilled, and the kingdom of God is at hand: repent, and believe the gospel" (Mark 1:15).

RIGHT NOW! How glorious is that? But the impact of "right now" only kicks in if we WILL repent and believe the gospel. In the scriptures we see where a father lays down his unbelief at the feet of Jesus, and his son is healed. That can happen for us TODAY.

In Mark 9:17-19, we can read the whole story. You might consider reading that if you want to actually walk in victory instead of just thinking about it.

The father tells Jesus that he took his afflicted son to the disciples, but they were not able to cast out the demons controlling him. Jesus exclaims, "O faithless generation, how long shall I be with you? Bring Him to me." He was trying to equip the disciples to do what He could do, because they were not there yet. After the healing, they asked Him why they themselves had been unsuccessful.

Here we are confronted with what many in the church today experience, which lead to statements like, "Well, sometimes God acts and sometimes He doesn't." The disciples were living with Jesus! They knew that wasn't true! Jesus tells them, "This kind can come forth by nothing but by prayer and fasting" (v. 29).

Moe and I heard a marvelous teaching on this recently that gave us a huge new insight. The words "this kind" was not about the demons, but about the BELIEF. We know that God has given us all the measure of faith we need. The demons are a defeated foe. The job has already been done on the cross. What needs to change is our belief.

Fasting and prayer help us tell our flesh and our emotions WHO is in charge. Sometimes the evidence of our senses, emotions, and intellect can be roadblocks to our belief, and we have to discipline them to come into perfect compliance with the Word of God.

Fasting and prayer do not move "demons" or any work of evil, including illness, and they do not move God. God is the same yesterday, today and forever. They are to move US. Fasting and prayer get our bodies and minds under control so that our BELIEF lines up with the belief of Jesus.

These spiritual exercises, performed on our bodies and minds, give us an opportunity to repent and believe the gospel, as Jesus exhorts us in Mark 1:14. This is Jesus speaking instructions for healing that will work for all mankind.

If we heed Jesus, repent, and believe the gospel, we will find that the kingdom of heaven is indeed at hand, right here and right now, just like He said!

Healing—A Little Adjustment

Sometime a little adjustment can make a big difference.

Recently, I was experiencing some discomfort in a part of my body that women watch carefully, because pain in that place can trigger fear and worse. But not in me, thank you. When fear knocks on my door, nobody answers! It turns out I was wearing the wrong size in a certain garment. Alleluia, was I happy it was a little thing like that! The adjustment was made, and ALL of me is very happy today!

It may be that what is necessary for health or healing may not be medical or spiritual warfare, but just an adjustment in lifestyle, attitude, nutrition, forgiveness or even underwear.

Scripture frequently reminds us of the importance of paying attention to the little things.

"A little that a righteous man has is better than the riches of many wicked" (Ps. 37:16).

"...a little sleep, a little slumber, a little folding of the hands: so shall your poverty come..." (Proverbs 6:10-11).

"Don't you know that a little leavening **leavens the whole loaf?**" (I Cor. 5:6).

"Even so, the tongue is a little member and boasts great things. Behold how great a matter a little fire kindles!" (James 3:5).

Remember the story of the widow's mite?

"Now Jesus sat opposite the treasury and saw how the people put money into the treasury. And many *who were* rich put in much. Then one poor widow came and threw in two mites, which make a quadrans. So He called His disciples to *Himself* and said to them, 'Assuredly, I say to you that this poor widow has put in more than all those who have given to the treasury; for they all put in out of their abundance, but she out of her poverty put in all that she had, her whole livelihood.'" (Mark 12:41-44)

"Father, we ask you to reveal the little thing that is standing in our way. Help us to see the small adjustments we need to make in order to discern what we need to do to be healed, be well, and most of all draw closer to you! Holy Spirit, thank you for the Still Small Voice, always available to us when we are available to listen. Jesus, you came to us as a tiny spark of life in a Virgin Mother's womb. Help us to remember, and to pay attention with reverence to the importance of little things. Amen."

Healing—Imagination

Can we agree that what we think about, dwell on, and stew over in our minds will have far greater manifestation in our lives than things we don't think about? That mental picture, repeated enough, can take hold and become a reality, either for awful or for wonderful results, such as pornography versus finding a cure for cancer.

Our imaginations are a powerful tool God has given us for a purpose. Obviously He intended it, as with all His gifts, to bring us joy. The gift and the joy were both corrupted right there in the garden, when at Satan's prompting Eve began to imagine what it would be like to know both good and evil. Thoughts and mental pictures held for long enough and strongly enough will eventually bear fruit.

This tool can make a critical difference in faith, especially faith for healing. The imagination can kick in 24/7/365 for good or ill unless we pay attention and take control over it before it takes control over us.

"And **God** saw that the wickedness of man was great in the earth, and that every imagining of the thoughts of his heart was only evil continually" (Genesis 6:5).

"...a heart that devises wicked imaginations, feet that be swift in running to mischief..." (Proverbs 6:18).

"For when they knew God, they neither glorified Him as God, nor were thankful, but became vain in their imaginations, and their foolish heart was darkened" (Romans 1:21).

"...who by the mouth of Thy servant David hast said, 'Why did the heathen rage, and the people imagine vain things?" (Acts 4:25).

...casting down imaginations, and every high thing that is exalted against the knowledge of God, and bringing every thought into captivity to the obedience of Christ... (II Corinthians 10:5).

Let's think on that last one a minute. Wow! The good news here is that we get to choose. We can CHOOSE what we will dwell on or what will manifest. We can bring EVERY thought and mental picture into agreement with God's wonderful plans and His wonderful imagination. We can refuse to build pictures of Satan's evil plans, and replace them with pictures of God's glorious plans for our lives.

That includes health and healing! Alleluia! Hot dog!

"Now to Him who is able to do exceedingly abundantly above all that we ask or imagine, according to the power that works in us, to Him be glory in the church by Christ Jesus to all generations, forever and ever. Amen" (Ephesians 3:20-21).

Healing—Who Is Taking the Lead?

Often we can't be led by God because we are too busy trying to lead Him. We can't hear what He's telling us we need to do because of the noise of us telling Him what to do. "My Way" may make a catchy song, but it certainly sounds puny next to God's way.

The worshiper in the 23rd Psalm tells us that God shepherds him...leads him...restores him...is with him...protects and saves him...feeds him...blesses him with goodness and mercy in this life and a home in the next. As my precious Hindu friend reminds me, voicing his summary of what Christians believe: "God has a plan!" That He does, but we must shut up and choose to walk in it.

I love that when the scripture tells us about Jesus healing people it includes examples of people who were maimed, deaf, dumb, and blind from birth. People try to limit what God can and will do with human qualifiers, "Well, that can't be healed because he was born with it." <u>News Flash: people are healed with infirmities they've had since birth</u>. Remember, God was the one who knit them together in their mother's womb.

"For you created my inmost being; you knit me together in my mother's womb" (Psalm 139:13).

Sometimes we are afraid to hope, hence the expression "hope against hope." Putting God in a box, deciding what He can or can't do or what He will or won't do is astonishing behavior for a Christian! We should know better than that! Falling into this is a good indicator that we are trying to lead God instead of God leading us.

Psalm 73:28 tells us that God's goodness is only limited by our capacity to receive it. II Chronicles 25:9 exhorts "God is able to give you much more than this!"

Maybe it's time to stop dancing around to our own tune and let God take the lead, without any instruction from us, and see what He will do as He keeps His promises!

Healing—Evidence of Things Seen!

Remember for a moment all the sweet pictures and statues you have seen over the years of the Good Shepherd. They tend to evoke messages of tenderness and love and protection and safety, and rightly so. Yet the sweetness can leave out the power that backs the tenderness.

In John 9 and 10, we read the story of the man born blind who is healed by Jesus. Instead of rejoicing, people questioned him and checked out the facts with his parents. They questioned whether Jesus is of God. The healing baffled them. People in our day can be baffled by healing too, afraid to claim it in faith, uneasy about seeking it, and afraid to call it a miracle to glorify God.

The formerly blind man clearly has received more than just physical sight! He teases the doubters (v. 30) and then points out that if Jesus were not from God, He could not have healed those eyes. Some accused Him of "having a devil," but others refuted this by replying, "Can a devil open the eyes of the blind?" (10:21).

Jesus explains the reality in an analogy of the work of a shepherd, which is decidedly more than posing for sweet pictures of Himself holding a lamb in His arms. He exhorts people, "If I do not the works of my father, believe me not. But if I do, though you don't believe me, believe the works: so you can know that the Father is in me and I in Him." (vs. 37-38) Jesus had no problem with healing being the convincing evidence rather than blind faith.

<u>It is amazing how a good controversy can distract us from the truth, and rob us of its power.</u>

In a recent discussion about how our lives can be transformed by walking in the power of God, one very highly intelligent and well-versed person commented, "Oh, I've heard this kind of teaching before." What kind would that be? The kind based on the Word? We tend to label each other, rejecting with a patronizing disdain those

"Word people" or those "Faith People" or those "Charismatic people" or those "fundamentalists"…or "those Catholics" and so on.

Me? I'm sticking with the blind man who wasn't blind any more. I'm believing in and counting on the One who could do the healing, the Good Shepherd who could kick the Devil's backside, and proved the power of God every place He went, and healed everyone. Want to label me? FINE! Label me the healed, the saved, the prosperous, the lamb in the arms of the Lamb who ain't afraid of nobody and certainly not of getting healed!

This Settles It

"These things I have spoken to you, that in Me you may have peace. In the world you will have tribulation; but be of good cheer, I have overcome the world" (John 16:33).

Four things that should solve all our life challenges, including sickness and disease and injury, are bluntly spoken in this one message:

1) **Jesus** said it.
2) He wants us to have peace.
3) Tribulation will be around trying to get at us.
4) He has overcome it.

"Quod erat demonstratum" for the logical. "Put that in your pipe and smoke it" for the hillbillies. "Well then, there y'a go" for the southern.

If you don't believe Jesus, I can't help you. If you won't embrace the promises of scripture, you are at the mercy of the world and all the tribulation out there.

Listen, if PEOPLE had the answers we'd have solved everything a long time ago! One wonderful discovery comes along and ten more diseases we've never heard of pop up.

Sometimes I just can't believe what I hear from BELIEVERS asking for healing prayer! You'd think we didn't know a thing and that God had either wanted us to suffer or kept the secret from us. That is blasphemy.

> There is no excuse for not being bullet proofed against illness.
> There is no room for doubt, confusion, or fear regarding illness.
> There is no excuse for standing helpless, as if you were helpless. You are not helpless.

Yes in this world it will come against us, **BUT...**

God wants you well.

He has told you so.

He has overcome the tribulation.
Evil is defeated. Good has won.

The bad stuff is out there, but we don't have to participate if we DO believe Jesus and we WILL believe the promises.

Arguing with me about this will be a serious waste of time, because I didn't make it up. God did, praise His holy name! Argue with GOD? Are you serious? Look what happened to that toothless dog Satan. He has no power! He just has to try and fool us into thinking he has some.

No, this thing has been settled once and for all. Take it or leave it.

I suggest you take it and start doing the overcoming Jesus has already won for you.

Q.E.D., there ya go!

A Thought Correction Away

Speaking of tribulation, I heard one of my favorite preachers say that tribulation has an expiration date. Don't you love that? It's like the old sour milk in the back of the fridge. Do you hang on to it, or do you throw it out? Therein lies the difference between extended misery and victory!

He also said that very often a breakthrough is just one thought correction away.

Let's assess the situation. God is all-powerful and loving, Jesus is Lord, the Holy Spirit is our Healer, and Satan is a defeated foe. The scripture references are in these healing messages. They are also in your Bible. So now we're clear on that.

True, the defeated foe is still roaming around, but he is "seeking whom he <u>may</u> devour." He can only mess with people who give Him permission (I Peter 5:8). We don't have to give it to him. If we give this truth a miss, we'll have to deal with the mess, because though defeated, our enemy is vigilant, and <u>we MUST be more diligent in believing what the Word promises than he is in denying it</u>.

Moe is always a "fruit inspector" in his life and in our home. If anything is not in accord with what the Word says we should have, speak, or do, he is ON IT! The first suspicion of discord, doubt, fear, accident, sickness and all the rest of it is recognized and dealt with immediately. We strive to catch them all early. It's easier to smash them when they are small, and we are constantly in prayer for the discernment we need. Should we fail, God is faithful!

It is important to recognize the signs that the enemy is looking for: envy, bitterness, lying, discord, fear, doubt, anger, sore this or that, "coming down with," ignorance, sin, accidents—in short, all the things that are contrary to the blessings God promises and wants us to have.

Let's commit to catch them small and stamp them out! Think seriously, because a breakthrough is sometimes only one though correction away.

What Will Make Us Whole?

Matthew Chapter 9 contains some straight talk from Jesus to the people He encountered while on the earth, and to us today.

We all recall the woman who received healing when she touched the hem of His garment in a crowd. He tells her (v. 22) that her FAITH has made her whole. He did not lay hands on her, or pray for her. There was nothing magical in that hem. The power was in her FAITH that He could heal and she could receive that healing.

In verses 28 and 29, two blind men request to receive their sight. Jesus asks them, "<u>Do you believe that I am able</u> to do this?" and they reply, "Yes, Lord." Then He touches their eyes and says, "<u>According to your faith be it unto you</u>," and they are healed.

According to my faith? Can it be that my faith plays a key part in all this? Apparently. This passage explained a lot to me! I realized I was getting the results I believed I'd get. Healing is not a question mark, and I had sometimes prayed for healing with a question mark "faith!"

I did not know what I did not know. That is the case with all of us! We find Jesus traveling to the cities and villages (v.35) teaching, preaching, and healing. Scripture says clearly that He healed EVERY sickness and EVERY disease!

We need teaching, preaching and healing today! When we search the scriptures for the truth, and learn under preachers and priests who proclaim the truth, we are strengthened to have the FAITH of that woman and the two blind men to believe what Jesus will do, and to receive it with joy.

We can walk in the whole peace, the shalom kind of peace, with nothing missing and nothing broken, if only we are willing to believe and be made whole.

Get Your Big "But" Out of the Way and Stop Slowing Down for Green Lights!

Did you ever notice those drivers who slow down for green lights? That baffles me! Yellow? Yes! Red? Of course, but **GREEN**? I don't get it. These are the fearful, who hesitate even for green lights.

Some people do this with their faith. Most of us have done it at one time or another. It often appears in the form of the word "but" following GOOD NEWS! "The tests came back negative, BUT...," "He said he thought he got it all in surgery, BUT....," "I believe that God can heal, BUT...," "I am not going to get sick, BUT...," "She continues to improve, BUT..." I'm not including what they say on the far side of the "BUT." We all know what it is! Sometimes they reverse the order. "We aren't out of the woods yet, BUT she's doing better."

Why are people so afraid to get out of the woods when they have the wood of the cross to settle it?

This happened in scripture, too. People are people! Check out Acts 4. When Peter and John and their guys were boldly marching through Georgia healing people left and right, the slow-down-for-green-lights crowd had objections! Look at what they said: "What shall we do to these men? A notable miracle had been done by them. That was clear to everyone who lived in Jerusalem; and they could not deny it, BUT so that it wouldn't spread any further among the people, they threatened them..."

Can you imagine? They ought to have rejoiced, praised God, brought everyone else sick or injured to be healed, and baked those good men pineapple upside down cakes!

BUT no-o-o-o-o!

However, most of them "glorified God for that which was done" (v.21). Those were the people who sailed happily right through the green lights. That should be us!

Yellow lights are good for caution, and red lights are critical for sin, but green lights mean "GO!" as every kindergarten child is taught.

Let's get our big BUTS out of the way once and for all. Let's fly when God gives us the green light of healing and glorify Him for what He has done!

The Whole Truth and Nothing But the Truth, So Help Me God

PROMISES:

If you diligently heed the voice of the **Lord** your God and do what is right in His sight, give ear to His commandments and keep all His statutes, I will put none of the diseases on you which I have brought on the Egyptians. For I *am* the **Lord** who heals you" (Exodus 15:26).

"For I *am* the **Lord**, I do not change; therefore you are not consumed..." (Malachi 3:6).

"In the world you will have tribulation; but be of good cheer, I have overcome the world" (John 16:33).

"You are of God, little children, and have overcome them, because He who is in you is greater than he who is in the world" (I John 4:4).

"For if, after they have escaped the pollutions of the world through the knowledge of the Lord and Savior Jesus Christ, they are again entangled in them and are overcome, the latter end is worse for them than the beginning" (II Peter 2:20).

God's great goodness is so vast and wonderful. Here are His promises, and a warning to keep us focused on them so that we can be whole: nothing missing, nothing broken. Think on these things.

The Dangers of Exposure

My parents often told me, laughing, that in my early, innocent youth I just loved EVERYBODY, without discrimination. They got tickled at the people who were not very lovable, watching their reactions to receiving that unconditional love.

As an adult, I struggle sometimes to love EVERYBODY like I did back then. After all, Jesus loves everybody. We're supposed to be like Him, and love everybody too. There is a very short list of people I'm still working to love, picturing them in my mind and heart as God sees them, as He created them to be. Then I can love them!

What does this have to do with healing? Well, although I love EVERYBODY, I can't afford to hang around with everybody if I want to get or stay healthy. Have you ever heard people say, "The best place to get sick is in a hospital with all those germs?" Ideas are even more contagious than germs, and more deadly.

I've discovered that my best bet is to be around faith filled people as much as possible, who refuse to think about, dwell on, fear and imagine illness, and instead focus on the will of God for health and healing.

It is so easy to get tired around tired people, discouraged around discouraged people, and sick around people who are always dwelling on illness. Note that sometimes those who are in a health battle are the most faith filled and inspiring people you can be around! So I'm not saying to avoid all of them! I know that if I join my faith with theirs in agreement with God's Word, both of us will be strengthened!

However, there are others who are always dwelling on sickness, who are suffering with something, all the time. They will be well informed, and eager to inform YOU of all the newest diseases and symptoms. They seem to define themselves by this, as if they have no value unless they have some ailment to complain about, worry about, think about, talk about, and they move through life from crisis to crisis.

We can pray for grace to fall on them and the joy of God's will for their health to catch them up into a new way of thinking, but in the meantime, we need to protect ourselves from too much exposure. We can't afford to allow the content of their imaginations to filter into our own thinking.

We must be steadfast in "...casting down imaginations, and every high thing that is exalted against the knowledge of God, and bringing every thought into captivity to the obedience of Christ" (II Cor. 10:5).

We are all cautious about exposing ourselves too much to certain things: sun, second hand smoke, insecticides, asbestos, and radon. We need to be equally careful about the imaginations we encounter as well. A powerful health measure may be to spend less time around some people and more time around others. That way we can still love EVERYONE!

The Power of Faith

Scriptures to support prayers for healing and health:

Bless the Lord, O my soul, and forget not all His benefits: who forgives all your iniquities; who heals all your diseases; who redeems your life from destruction; who crowns you with loving-kindness and tender mercies; who satisfies your mouth with good things; so that your youth is renewed like the eagle's" (Ps. 103:1-5).

"Jesus Christ the same yesterday, and today, and forever" (Hebrews 13:8).

"Heal me, O Lord, and I shall be healed; save me, and I shall be saved: for thou art my praise" (Jer. 17:14).

"For I will restore health to you, and I will heal you of your wounds, says the Lord" (Jer. 30:17).

"Do not be afraid, for I am with you: don't be dismayed; for I am your God: I will strengthen you; yes, I will help you, yes I will uphold you with the right hand of my righteousness" (Isaiah 41:10).

"He was wounded for our transgressions, He was bruised for our iniquities; the chastisement of our peace was upon Him; and with His stripes we are healed (Is. 53:5).

"And behold, there came a leper and worshipped Him saying, Lord if you will, you can make me clean. And Jesus put forth His hand, and touched him, saying I will, be clean. And immediately his leprosy was cleansed" (Matt.8:16-17).

"And all things whatsoever you ask in prayer, believing, you shall receive" (Matt. 21:22).

"And these signs shall follow those who believe: In my name they shall cast out devils; they shall speak with new tongues; they shall take up serpents; and if they drink any deadly thing, it shall not hurt them; they shall lay hands on the sick and they shall recover" (Mark 16:16-18).

"And the whole multitude sought to touch Him: for there went virtue out of Him, and healed them all" (Luke 6:19).

"There came also a multitude out of the cities around Jerusalem, bringing sick folks, and those who were vexed with unclean spirits: and they were healed every one" (Acts 5:16).

"But if the Spirit of Him that raised up Jesus from the dead dwell in you, He that raised up Christ from the dead shall also quicken your mortal bodies by His Spirit that dwells in you" (Romans 8:11).

"Is any sick among you? Let him call for the elders of the church: and let them pray over him, anointing him with oil in the name of the Lord: And the prayer of faith shall save the sick, and the Lord shall raise him up; and if he has committed sins they shall be forgiven him. Confess your faults to one another, and pray for one another, that you may be healed. The effective fervent prayer of a righteous man avails much" (James 5:14-16).

"Beloved, I wish above all things that you may prosper and be in good health, even as your soul prospers" (3 John: 2).

"Jesus Christ the same yesterday, and today, and forever." (Hebrews 13:8)

WEAPONS for Health and Healing

1) _____'s faith is the substance of things hoped for; the <u>evidence</u> of things not seen. (Heb. 11:1)
2) Jesus Himself took _____ infirmities and bore <u>his/her sickness</u>. (Matt. 8:17)
3) What things soever _____ asks, when he/she prays, believing that he/she receives them, <u>he/she shall have</u>. (Mark 11:24)
4) Jesus gave His apostles power and delegated authority over all devils, <u>and to cure diseases</u>—including_____'s! (Luke 9:1-2) They took that authority and "healed every where" (Luke 9:6)
5) Jesus said, "These signs shall follow <u>them that believe…</u>"…they shall lay hands on the sick, and <u>they shall recover</u>." (Mark 16:15-18)
6) Jesus said, "Behold, I give you power to tread on serpents and scorpions, and over ALL THE POWER OF THE ENEMY: and NOTHING shall by any means hurt you." (Luke 10:19)
7) Greater is He that is in _____, than he who is in the world. (John 4:4)
8) If _____ asks any thing in my name, I will do it. (John 14:13-14)
9) With His stripes _____ is healed…with His stripes _____ was healed. (Is. 53:5; I Peter 2:24)
10) Is _____ sick? Call for the elders of the church and let them pray for him/her, anointing him/her with oil in the name of the Lord: and the <u>prayer of faith shall save him/her</u>, and <u>the Lord will raise him/her up</u>. (James 5:14-15)
11) Jesus bore _____'s sicknesses <u>for him/her</u>! (Matt. 8:17)
12) _____ shall come to <i>his/her grave in a full age like a shock of corn comes in its season</i> (Job 5:26) after living a fruitful life (Ps. 92:14) fulfilling the number of his/her days (Ex. 23:26) until he/she shall be forever with the Lord (I Thess. 4:17).

13) *"Because _____has set his/her love upon me, therefore I will deliver him/her: I will set him/her on high, because he/she has known my name. He/she shall call upon me, and I will answer him/her: I will be with him/her in trouble; I will deliver him/her, and honor him/her. With long life I will satisfy him/her, and show him/her my salvation." (Ps. 91:14-16)*

14) *"My covenant with _____I will not break, nor alter the thing that has gone out of my lips." (Ps. 89:34)*

15) *Jesus Christ the same yesterday, and today, and forever!* **(Heb.3:8)**

John 17—Get Real!

One of our healing prayer team, Monica from Georgia, mentioned to me recently how even believers miss the benefits of the Christian life by "picking and choosing" scriptures to live by. The irony, she pointed out, is not that they choose to ignore the scriptures about avoiding their favorite sins...it is that they also choose sometimes to ignore the scriptures about wonderful blessings like healing, prosperity, and happiness!

Beware: If the enemy can't trip you up with evil, he'll try to trip you up with good! How? By convincing you that you have no right to expect it. That you have to be "realistic." I don't know about you, but the fallen world's "realism" has no appeal for me. I'd rather live in God's reality.

The entire chapter of John 17 includes a conversation Jesus, God the Son, has with God the Father. He is getting ready to leave the earth, knowing the Holy Spirit will soon be indwelling in people here in this life. He has set the example of how we are to live, and how we can live. He has performed miracles continuously, and demonstrated the power of love. He mentions one by one all the things He has given us and revealed to us, including our unity with Him. Heaven says, "I am glorified in them." Jesus is glorified in us!

Well, yes, but only when we are living the gifts and the revelation.

1) "And now I come to thee: and these things I speak in the world, that they might have my joy fulfilled in themselves. I have given them thy word..." (vs.13-14) and

2) "They are not of the world even as I am not of the world. Sanctify them through thy truth. Thy word is truth." (vs. 16-17)

Living in this powerful reality is the option we have, offered freely by our loving Father. He will not force us to choose it. We can be saved and still choose to walk in sickness, financial lack, and stress. Let's be honest and clear, however: those are not God's will for us.

They are the enemy's lies, and he is the defeated foe, unless we hand him back his power.

That's the reality, there in red letters in Chapter 17. I don't know about you, but I'm up for getting real God's way!

Healing—Use the Show Towels!

Why are people, even BELIEVERS, sometimes hesitant or reluctant to receive God's best gifts? As I was pondering this, I remembered the story of The Show Towels.

Friends were visiting us for a few days. The first night, the husband headed for the shower, and called down to me, "Sharon, where can I find some towels?"

I called back, "Aaron, they are hanging in your bathroom."

He then asked, "But aren't these the SHOW TOWELS?"

I'd never heard of show towels! I assured him that those towels were for him, and he was welcome to use them. On another occasion, when another couple was visiting, they used one hand towel only, and shared it between the two of them. They said they didn't want to use those nice towels!

We all got a big laugh over this. I explained that all my towels were there to be used. Don't look around for raggedy towels or drip dry when I have provided perfectly good towels for your drying pleasure!

But there is more to this story. When sharing it with my mother, who also thought it was funny, she remarked, "Maybe they meant the COMPANY towels." Oh. Yes. In our house we did always pull out the newer towels for the company, to give them the best we had. The reason was not for "show" but for honor.

When it comes to God's best gifts for us, like healing, are we deceived into thinking that they are not for us? Do we leave the miracles hanging on the rack, thinking they are just "for show" and not for use? God's deepest desire is to give us, His beloved children, His best, not for show and not because we are company, but because He loves us. His gifts are not shabby or raggedy, they are abundant and glorious and all for us!

Have you ever seen the film *Chariots of Fire*?[6] If not, I recommend it. At a key moment in this true story, someone gives a godly runner in the Olympics a note which quotes the verse from I Samuel 2:30: "For those who honor me I will honor."

That is the will of God's heart, from towels to healing to every good gift. Receive it! Our worthiness has nothing to do with it. His gifts are never just for show. Snatch them off the racks, and use your show towels today! Remember that in God's house, His family gets the very best.

Healing—The Great God of Little Things

Have you ever noticed how often people wait to seek God's help? They wait until a little symptom, a little pain, a little test grows, until mixed with fear and anxiety, it turns into something huge and *then* they cry out for a miracle?

Of course God is the God of HUGE. Nothing is huge to Him. Hideous disease is as easily destroyed by Him as you and I would eat a Popsicle. No size or strength will ever impress God. He MADE huge! Miracles are common for Him, and He desires that they become common for us, as we trust Him more and more.

"Behold, the nations are as a drop in a bucket, And are counted as the small dust on the scales; Look, He lifts up the isles as a very little thing" (Is. 40:15).

So what is this tendency to try to fix the small things ourselves instead of going to Him immediately? He is also the God of SMALL things! Every little scraped knee, sore toe, rash, fever, growth, cough, lump and bump is as important to Him as a full-fledged, raging disease. It is not necessary for us to be baffled, at our wits end, and terrified before we ask, "God, would you fix this?"

"Do you not know that a little leaven leavens the whole lump? " (I Cor. 5:6).

It may be that our awe in the wonder of His vastness distracts us from the tenderness of His concern for even the smallest events in our lives. He cares about every little thing. When we get through throwing a fit and wailing and carrying on...when we calm down and quietly ask for His help, His answer will be loving and gentle:

"...and after the earthquake a fire, but the Lord was not in the fire; and after the fire a still small voice" (I Kings 19:12).

He will answer every time, the big things, yes...but the little things as well.

Get Busy—All Shook Up

This morning God put a question on my heart: "What do you think my people could be doing if they weren't so busy being sick?"

That question shook me up. Remember the Elvis song, "All Shook Up?" This was about romantic love, and there is quite an ad on TV recently using it very effectively! The key line in it is "I'm in love...I'm all shook up."

God is in love with us, and I'm in love with Him, and I AM all shook up when He reveals things to me like this question today. What WOULD we be doing if we were not so busy being...

Sick
Worried
Fearful
Tired
Discouraged
Sinful
Broke

Busted and Disgusted?

God has provided us antidotes to all of these things that can become strongholds in our lives, taking up the valuable time He intended to dwell in His peace and love and accomplish the things He created us to do during our time in the flesh on this earth.

"These things I have spoken to you, that in Me you may have peace. In the world you will[a] have tribulation; but be of good cheer, I have overcome the world" (John 16:33).

In trying to support friends going through financial issues recently, it surprised us that they were very closed-minded to solutions, stuck on the problem, blind to the solution! A mutual friend commented in frustration, "They are so busy being broke that they won't take time to get out of debt."

If we're not careful, we can get stuck too in issues of health and everything else on the bad list. God has provided us the way to get unstuck, if we'll start spending our time on the right thing!

> "So too the (Holy) Spirit comes to our aid and bears us up in our weakness; for we do not know what prayer to offer...but the Spirit Himself...pleads in our behalf with unspeakable yearnings and groanings too deep for utterance."—Romans 8:26

"Thank you, dear Father and Lord of my life, for the question you asked me today. You have answered it for me. I can see all the things I can do in you. I know I can do them, because I'm in Love, and I'm all shook up."

Pay Attention = Good Cheer!

Are you a person who pays attention to what is going on in THE world and not just YOUR world? I strongly believe that we should do this, because although we are not "of" the world, we are IN IT by the will of God for a purpose, and therefore need to be aware.

In times like these, that can be worrisome until we remember that God is in charge, Jesus has overcome the world, and the Holy Spirit will direct us if we'll just listen and obey. That snaps me back into perspective immediately, and I can be the cheerful person He made me to be!

I was checking out the "In this world you will have tribulation; but be of good cheer, I have overcome the world (John 16:32-33)" scripture and to my delight found lots more!

Matthew 9:2

"Then behold, they brought to Him a paralytic lying on a bed. When Jesus saw their faith, He said to the paralytic, "Son, be of good cheer; your sins are forgiven you."

Matthew 9:22

"But Jesus turned around, and when He saw her He said, 'Be of good cheer, daughter; your faith has made you well.' And the woman was made well from that hour."

Matthew 14:27

"But immediately Jesus spoke to them, saying, 'Be of good cheer! It is I; do not be afraid.'"

Mark 6:50

"..for they all saw Him and were troubled. But immediately He talked with them and said to them, 'Be of good cheer! It is I; do not be afraid.'"

Mark 10:49

"So Jesus stood still and commanded him to be called. Then they called the blind man, saying to him, 'Be of good cheer. Rise, He is calling you.'"

Luke 8:48

"And He said to her, 'Daughter, be of good cheer; your faith has made you well. Go in peace.'"

So, when we are paying attention to all the nonsense that is going on out there, we can just laugh and stay cheerful and powerful!

Here we see that our sins are forgiven, our faith can make us well, He is with us always so we don't need to be afraid, He is calling us, and we can go in peace! We can laugh at tribulation!

Don't you just know the devil hates that?

Healing—Spirit Spell Check

Do you have that Spell-check feature on your home computer or other device? It is such a terrific help, but it does have its limitations when it tries to re-spell a word it does not recognize. I get a kick out of the way it re-names some of my friends!

Many people have this feature, but still have miserable spelling in their documents because:

1) they don't know it's there
2) don't know how to use it
3) have turned it off
4) ignore it

The Holy Spirit can be ignored in the same way, and He is full of corrections that can heal us and keep us well, but some people don't know He's there, don't know how to use Him, have turned Him off, or ignore Him.

This is foolish for our good friend Spell-check and tragically dangerous for our best friend the Holy Spirit. Neither will work. Both are available and ready to help if recognized, used, kept on at all times, and always receiving our attention.

Sometimes even Spell-check doesn't get it! Spelling is tricky, think "meet" and "meat" for example. Both are spelled just fine, but if used in the wrong context can still be wrong. If it does not know your name, such as Ghassami, it will try to re-name you!

The Holy Spirit knows exactly how to spell your name, and to lead you into the wonderful life God has planned for you. All the subtle differences the enemy can throw at you can be immediately checked and corrected!

No circumstance in life can re-name you. God created us each with a unique nature and a special purpose in mind. We are privileged to always:

1) Know He is there
2) Learn how to use His gifts
3) Keep our receiver turned on
4) Abide in Him forever

Precautionary Measures

Precautionary measures! How often we are warned to take them in advance of potential inconvenience, danger, or disaster. We learn to look both ways before we cross the street, to brush our teeth after every meal, to get an annual physical, and to eat fruits and vegetables.

Scripture gives us powerful tips to prevent disaster in many areas of human life, including prevention of illness, injury, and suffering. Have you noticed that there are times when you are asked to pray for lots of people who seem to have come down with some bug at the same time? Has it seemed at times that one particular disease appears to be causing tremendous crisis in the lives of multiple people? Does it ever strike you that certain families seem to always have some medical crisis going on? One gets solved and two more pop up? Back on the prayer list again?

Like the Girl Scouts, we would do well to "Be Prepared" at all times! Proverbs 13 impresses upon us: "The law of the wise is a fountain of life, to depart from the snares of death. Whoever despises the word shall be destroyed: but he who fears the commandments shall be rewarded" (vs 13-14).

The Girl Scout manual taught me to be prepared; the Word of God is the manual of serious believers. Searching the Word for precautionary measures IN ADVANCE will bullet proof, fire proof, and disaster proof us better than any other means available in this life. With their direction, we can look both ways when crossing the streets of life, depart from the snares of death, and live.

Who Is in Control?

We humans are spirits who have a mind and live in a body, hence the phrase "spirit, soul, and body." The eternal spirit, when in harmony with the Holy Spirit of God, is the ultimate in safety, health, joy, and all good and glorious things so desired for us and gifted to us by our creator and heavenly father.

Sometimes the three come into conflict, which can prevent us from receiving the healing power of God. Have you heard, "The spirit is willing but the flesh is weak?" (Mark 14:38). When our flesh or our minds are in control, then our healing is dependent on how strong we are physically or how smart we, or some other person, may be.

God gave us the answer to this situation in Psalm 119:105: "Thy word is a lamp unto my feet and a light unto my path." It is His wisdom that will provide the light to illuminate the way we need to go to avoid stumbling during our time on earth in the flesh.

This Word is a real power, the highest power! It penetrates into every aspect of the human being—spirit, soul and body—and provides a check on whether our thoughts and beliefs are in agreement with God: Hebrews 4:12 "For the word of God is alive and active. Sharper than any double-edged sword, it penetrates even to dividing soul and spirit, joints and marrow; it judges the thoughts and attitudes of the heart."

That is something to wrap your mind around, isn't it? Once grasped, however, what glorious peace we can have in the knowledge that God's eternal wisdom had been given to us.

I Peter 1:25 says, "All Flesh is like grass, and its glory like the flower of grass. The grass withers, and the flower falls off, but the word of the Lord endures forever. And this is the word which was preached to you."

Isaiah 40:8: "The grass withers and the flowers fall, but the word of our God endures forever."

Glory! Isn't That Just the Most Amazing Thing?

We have a responsibility to our flesh and to our testimony as followers of Jesus the Christ:

Hebrews 6:4-6 says, "For it is impossible for those who were once enlightened, and have tasted the heavenly gift, and have become partakers of the Holy Spirit, and have tasted the good word of God and the powers of the age to come, if they fall away, to renew them again to repentance, since they crucify again for themselves the Son of God, and put Him to an open shame."

With God's help, and the revelation revealed to us in His Word, we can live lives filled with His power and goodness and health and peace in every aspect of our being: spirit, soul, and body! Alleluia! What a Savior!

Voice Recognition

"Behold I stand at the door and knock: if any man hears my voice and opens the door, I will come in to him, and will sup with him and he with me" (Revelation 3:20).

Hearing from God is the most important skill we can possibly attain in this life on earth, wouldn't you agree? Have you ever been in a situation where you really needed to know what to say or do, and wished you could sit down with Jesus and ask Him? Well you can! If Revelation 3:20 is to be believed, He is waiting for you to open the door. He has already knocked!

"How do you know it's from God?" people ask. Well how do you recognize the voice of anyone you know? Your Mom or Dad, your beloved spouse, or your cherished child? You don't have to ask if the voice belongs to them, you know it, and know it well. We know that infants learn to recognize the voice of their mothers and fathers in the womb.

There are lots of voices out there competing for our attention. We hear our own, and those of people from the past, true voices and false voices. The voice of God is unmistakable. So, how do we learn it?

We have a dear friend who is on a learning curve about Christianity. He has been informing people that they are going to hell. Sometimes this is the right thing to do, but sometimes it is NOT, and can drive them away rather than toward the redeeming, healing love of God. These announcements of his have been disastrous! A good tip for him would be to remember the sound of whatever voice prompted him to do that, and label that one "NOT GOD!"

When we make a conscious choice to do disastrous, destructive, stupid, hurtful, idiotic things we can be sure that the voice we were hearing to egg us on was NOT the voice of God!

"You will seek me and find me when you search for me with your whole heart," the Lord in Jeremiah 29:13 assures and promises us.

One moment in time, you suddenly hear Him. Hear, perceive, sense, experience, whatever one can say to describe such an event.

When that happens, you KNOW who it is! That is, if you are paying attention. You can note the unmistakable difference in that Voice, and you will begin to hear it more and more.

After knowing reality, many people experience a, "I could have had a V-8" moment. They realize that God has spoken to them before, but they thought it was just a brilliant idea out of their own mind. All glorious inspiration, sudden perceptions of truth we will eventually recognize as moments with the ultimate Creator.

We can be brilliant, but not *that* brilliant! Once we recognize that Voice over and over because we are listening for it and answering the knock on the door, we can be brilliant *all* the time.

Listen and Live!

The "Voice Recognition" message was a set up for this one. God has really been working on me about this subject, and I'm paying attention!

Hearing from God is the ultimate in disease, injury, and disaster prevention, as well as in what to do when an unexpected crisis hits.

"If any of you lacks wisdom, let him ask of God, who gives to all liberally and without reproach, and it will be given to him."(James 1:5)

Day by day, moment by moment God is speaking to us. The Holy Spirit is constantly there, available for consultation. We can be prompted:

Don't eat that. (It will upset your stomach.)

Avoid touching these apples. (Someone with a disease has just infected them.)

Stick that burned hand under cold water and pray. (Your obedience will open the door to immediate healing.)

Do not attend that event. (Conversation that will take place there will put doubt in the minds of your children.)

Go to the doctor or don't go. (I will use him/witness to him or he does not know how to help you with this. I have revealed to him how to help you.)

Take a different route in the car today. (You will avoid an accident.)

You need to be taking a daily vitamin. You need to change the vitamin you are taking. (Your body is missing some important nutrition. You need to take a more effective supplement.)

Go out into the sun/come in out of the sun. (You are getting too little/too much.)

Do not send you child to that play date. (Avoid being exposed to meningitis.)

Once you have learned to recognize God's voice, and commit to hearing and obeying, your vulnerability is vastly decreased, as is the time you are now possibly putting into research from dozens of other sources. Do you really think another source will give you better information than God? "For the wisdom of this world is foolishness with God" (1 Corinthians 3:19).

Of course sometimes He prompts us to seek out wisdom from another person, book, internet site, etc., but all too often we go out half-cocked on our own and waste time or miss the true solution, and instead delay or act on false options that will lead us in the wrong direction.

"Does not their own excellence go away? They die, even without wisdom" (Job 4:21).

Sadly, I have recently heard of many attacks by a particular disease, and in my spirit I felt the knowledge that these could have been avoided and could be healed, if people would only listen to our Heavenly Father.

"Therefore, behold, I will again do a marvelous work among this people, a marvelous work and a wonder; for the wisdom of their wise men shall perish, and the understanding of their prudent men shall be hidden" (Isaiah 29:14).

Are you tempted to think, "Oh, Sharon you're being too simplistic! It's not that simple!" <u>Oh, yes it is!</u> It's much simpler than walking through life blindly, vulnerable to all the pain and suffering Jesus died on the cross to vanquish. The same God who just told me what you might be thinking can tell you that.

"Wisdom is the principal thing; therefore get wisdom and in all your getting, get understanding" (Proverbs 4:7).

In other words, listen up!

You and DIFFERENT

Did you ever become annoyed, indignant, or outraged when you heard someone you know well being totally misrepresented? Did you adamantly insist that is was NOT an accurate picture of how she or he behaved?

God is misrepresented more than any of the finest people we know, and sometimes by His own people, who out of ignorance represent Him as if He were a powerless or heartless human being.

The Lord goes out of His way in scripture to let us know that if we come to HIM, our case is different! There is a HUGE difference in whether you choose to belong to Him or not. Is there a difference in being a Christian vs. any other faith? YES! In both the Old and New Testaments, God makes it clear that there are enormous advantages in being a person who chooses to trust all of life to Him, to seek His guidance and protection, and to walk in the light of His path. He created everyone out of His unfailing love, and wants everyone to receive His best gifts as beloved children. However, each of us has an individual free choice. If we choose Him, the benefits kick in: He will...

..call His servants by another name;

"So that he who blesses himself in the earth shall bless himself in the God of truth; And he who swears in the earth shall swear by the God of truth; because the former troubles are forgotten, and because they are hidden from My eyes" (Is. 65:16).

Also, contrary to what you often hear, He does not hide His wisdom from us, but reveals it FOR our benefit:

"... that their hearts may be encouraged, being knit together in love, and attaining to all riches of the full assurance of understanding, to the knowledge of the mystery of God, both of the Father and of Christ, in whom are hidden all the treasures of wisdom and knowledge" (Col. 2:2-3).

Paul admonishes, "... I became a minister according to the stewardship from God, which was given to me for you, to fulfill the word of God the mystery, which has been hidden from ages and from generations, but now has been revealed to His saints. To them God willed to make known what are the riches of the glory of this mystery among the Gentiles, which[a] is Christ in you, the hope of glory" (Col. 1:25-27).

Contrary to the slander we so often hear—slander that misleads people into believing that God wants us to suffer helplessly—our God does not tease us by withholding key information, keeping secret the vital information that would help us to overcome the tribulations of this world.

No, when we choose Him, we get it all! Every promise, every help, every gift, and every good thing! Isn't that what we want for our own children? Are we better parents than God? We should be outraged at the very idea! Let's fight the slander we hear all around us, and sometimes in our own hearts, and instead embrace the reality: because of His love, when we choose Him He will prove to us in every way that WE ARE DIFFERENT.

Can You Afford That?

One of the dearest, most respected women who had changed my life through her godly wisdom once remarked that she was more careful with spiritual choices than material ones. She had learned the scriptural lessons concerning material prosperity, followed them, and had become a great example of the wealth that comes from obeying God's guidelines. She said it was amazing to learn that she was very materialistic when she had too little and not materialistic at all when she had plenty to share.

She then turned to sickness and disease/health and wellness, eager to learn how to make the same life change in that aspect of her life, and got BINGO! Again! The key in any area where you have a need is to ask the question when making choices, "Can I afford that?" We are not asking in terms of money so much as in terms of your mind and your spirit.

My mother used to nix certain movies for her kids, saying, "No, that one's too googy!" "Too googy" must be a mom industry term. It meant too scary, too dark, or too evil. She and my dad did not want their children to have fear, even in entertainment. All of us loved murder mysteries if they were in the manner of the Golden Age of mystery writing, wherein good and evil were at odds, and good always won in the end. What Mom objected to was a film that generated feelings of fear or horror. She said we could not afford to fill our minds and hearts with "googy" because that led to nightmares, and God has not given us a spirit of fear.

Applying that wisdom from two beloved wise women in my life, I learned to examine the resources I trust very carefully. On one occasion, something was "going on" in my body. I asked a bunch of people who filled me with horror stories, read up on symptoms, etc. You know, there is always a boatload of bad news out there if you make yourself vulnerable. In the middle of all that brilliant investigation, at a friend's suggestion I picked up my Bible to see what God had to say about my situation.

BINGO! In minutes the fear left me. In an hour the symptoms abated. In a week I was totally fine. Every time I go for a check up, that issue never comes up, AND I DON'T BRING IT UP. I realized that I can't afford some things:

1) The kind of investigation that leads to deeper and deeper panic
2) The seeking conversation with people who love to tell horror stories
3) Reliance on any power or authority over that of Almighty God
4) Looking for trouble just in case it's there

Why? I've realized <u>I can't afford it</u> if I want to be healthy!

Indeed, God has prompted me on occasion to speak to my doctor, change my vitamins, eat something, or cut something out of my diet.

The cost of consulting God is simply love, attention, submission and gratitude. The cost of consulting any other source first is too expensive: we can't afford it!

Matthew 11:28-30: "Come to Me, all you who labor and are heavy laden, and I will give you rest. Take My yoke upon you and learn from Me, for I am gentle and lowly in heart, and you will find rest for your souls. For My yoke is easy and My burden is light."

Bit Him

This past week I had a funny healing! Last time I was at the dentist he took x-rays clearly revealing that I needed work to remove a large cavity formed in an inconvenient place between two teeth, requiring two crowns and lots of money. Well OK, I thanked God that we had the money to pay for them. Moe, however, laid his hands on me every night and claimed healing for the cavity.

Then I went back, and the dentist took new x-rays. No cavity! Can you believe it? YES is the answer. I should have known better, but I said, "Golly, I didn't know it would work for TEETH!" Moe reminded me that <u>it will work for everything</u>.

We shared this in church one Sunday, and our deacon remarked that it works for everything but you must have faith, a modest statement but a critical and powerful one. Even I, your humble healing correspondent, would have missed it this time if Moe hadn't exercised his authority over his household and expected healing for me.

Bit by bit, from faith to faith, we grow toward the Truth set before us. When we pray for healing, if that is exactly what we EXPECT. He is that kind of God!

The enemy lost that round because of Moe's faith and God's faithfulness. I have the teeth to bite him back. That's what we need, isn't it? Faith with teeth!

Faith Facing Facts

On the heels of "faith with teeth in it," let's take a look at those faith teeth again. When it comes to sickness and disease in scripture, there is incontrovertible evidence that these are EVIL. They are to be avoided and they are identified on the dark side of the fall, not God's will, but man's consequences.

For centuries, people had no problem calling evil accurately. Even today many people, and most children, can identify it for what it is. However, there is a tendency to explain away wrong behavior, bad choices, and disastrous consequences by renaming them something other than what they are. Often criminal behavior is renamed some kind of illness. WHY? Because <u>illness is no longer seen as evil</u>.

On occasion, most of us have probably informed the TV that calling crime a sickness is so wrong that it is dangerous. However, we shy away from getting angry about sickness and disease being accepted as a normal part of life. We SHOULD BE FURIOUS! You'd rip the head off of a predator approaching your little daughter, but if the flu threatens, do you just placidly accept it as "Oh well, there's a lot of that going around."

Controversial? You bet. Jesus was the most controversial person who walked the earth, and what did He do? He demonstrated that sickness was EVIL, and got rid of it. Why is this so hard for us to understand? Because we get lots of help from our enemy who wants to keep us distracted and confused…and sick.

Notice how often Jesus paired reference to sins being forgiven when He performed healings?

"Some men brought to Him a paralyzed man, lying on a mat. When Jesus saw their faith, He said to the man, "Take heart, son; your sins are forgiven" (Matthew 9:2).

"When Jesus saw their faith, He said to the paralyzed man, "Son, your sins are forgiven" (Mark 2:5).

"Which is easier: to say to this paralyzed man, 'Your sins are forgiven,' or to say, 'Get up, take your mat and walk'?" (Mark 2:9).

"When Jesus saw their faith He said, Friend, your sins are forgiven" (Luke 5:20).

Clearly in pairing sin and sickness as evils He can vanquish, He makes it difficult to avoid facing facts: both are evil, and both can be overcome by His power and love.

ALL THINGS contrary to the will of God for us are WRONG and EVIL, and we should not have to put up with them. The good news is that we don't have to keep sinning. The good news is also that we don't have to keep getting sick.

We live in a world and a culture that often seems to have diminished or ignored the power of evil, renaming it and distracting us from the facts. Don't be duped another day of your life. The reality is that Jesus came to forgive sins and to heal. Take up your faith to face the facts, and live.

How to Handle the Bully

Probably all of us watch the film "A Christmas Story" at least once every holiday season. One of the best scenes involves Ralphie facing and defeating the bully Farkus. In earlier scenes we see this bully making life miserable in a variety of ways for many kids, including his own sidekick in intimidation. One day, Ralphie has had enough, and Farkus is totally vanquished.

Our Bully has been totally vanquished too! Jesus had him truly beaten on the cross. However, he will still wander the earth seeking anyone he can trick (1 Peter 5:8), "Be sober, be vigilant; because your adversary the devil walks about like a roaring lion, seeking whom he may devour." We can be fooled or distracted or frightened or exhausted into allowing this defeated foe to bully us once again if we're not careful.

We need to work vigilantly to remind our flesh and our minds and our hearts that evil has NO right to us, period. We may be making headway where it comes to sin, how are we doing with sickness and disease? The same fervency that "has had enough" like Ralphie when it comes to sin can have the same fervency with sickness! Satan does not want us to remember that. He, and we, are reminded of that throughout scripture:

"Then Jesus said to Him, Away with you, Satan! For it is written, 'You shall worship the **Lord** your God, and Him only you shall serve'" (Matthew 4:10). We do NOT have to go along with his evil designs over us, spirit, soul OR body. We can follow the example of Jesus and <u>CAST HIM OUT</u>. Jesus set this example so many times, how can we possibly miss it?

"But He turned and said to Peter, "Get behind Me, Satan! You are an offense to me, for you are not mindful of the things of God, but the things of men" (Matthew 16:23). Allowing Satan's will rather than God's in any aspect of our being is the result of thinking like people think instead of thinking like God. People think sometimes nothing can be done for us if the doctor can't cure it. Do you really think God is limited by what the doctor can't cure?

"And He was there in the wilderness forty days, tempted by Satan, and was with the wild beasts; and the angels ministered to Him." Jesus was in a difficult and uncomfortable situation, and God provided help for Him! Our angels are at the ready to aid us too!

"And these are the ones by the wayside where the word is sown. When they hear, Satan comes immediately and takes away the word that was sown in their hearts (Mark 4:15). We can understand our rights as redeemed children of God, yet forget them in an instant of pain or a bad report.

Jesus was tempted by Satan, but He had help, "Then Jesus, being filled with the Holy Spirit, returned from the Jordan and was led by the Spirit into the wilderness" (Luke 4:1). The Holy Spirit was sent to mankind at Pentecost to be our protector and advocate, our teacher, and guide, but so often people just wear red on Pentecost Sunday and never embrace the benefits of His power and love. He IS GOD, yet He is ignored.

"So ought not this woman, being a daughter of Abraham, whom Satan has bound for eighteen years, be loosed from this bond on the Sabbath?" (Luke 13:16). Think about it. Eighteen years she was bound. It is perfectly clear in scripture that no matter how long a person has suffered, he or she can be healed! Some people were born with an infirmity, and Jesus healed them. Others suffered many years, like the woman with the issue of blood. That's nothing to God! How hideous to think that just because you've suffered a long time it means God wants it that way!

"...to open their eyes, in order to turn them from darkness to light, and from the power of Satan to God, that they may receive forgiveness of sins and an inheritance among those who are sanctified by faith in Me" (Acts 26:18). At any moment, at any time, we can walk out of the darkness and into the light of God's forgiving, healing grace. Ralphie realized in a moment that he did not have to take the bullying any more, and he settled it right there on the playground. Everyone saw it. The bully was exposed, weakened and defeated.

"And the God of peace will crush Satan under your feet shortly. The grace of our Lord Jesus Christ be with you. Amen" (Romans 16:20).

I am weeping, and my heart is on fire as I read this wonderful closing word from God to each of us. We live after the crushing has been done. If we truly receive God's promise, the bully can't hurt us any more.

When Will You Have the Time to Get Healed?

There are so many truly good things we can do with our time. They are not frivolous or sinful things, they're good things. We can shuttle kids around, enjoy fun times with friends, go to a game or watch a movie, get a massage or a pedicure, support a charity, absorb ourselves in work, and fulfill all our obligations to so many people.

When will you find time to get healed?

We humans are interesting. We can be very high maintenance, and very self-absorbed. Just when do we find time to focus on the victory Jesus has won for us? How bad does the pain have to get? How often have you known someone, maybe a really wonderful person, happily moving through life until sickness takes hold and begins to take over? Attention to other aspects of life diminishes as the pain increases. More and more time is spent on seeking solutions.

At some point, when none of these avenues solves the problem, the person turns to God. Maybe it is to question Him, or to plead with Him, or to blame Him.

Now they start comparing themselves with Job! Then they start wondering if their suffering is somehow part of God's plan. They start believing that they must "suffer with Him."

Does this sound familiar?

God's will is clear. He never told anyone to go suffer. He sent Jesus, who trained His disciples in what they were to do, by setting the example Himself. Remember, He had set aside His divine powers to walk as a man on this earth to show us how to live. Don't we get all holy sometimes and say, "Oh, I just want to be more like Jesus"? What would that mean? Well, here you go:

"...preach the gospel to the poor, heal the brokenhearted, preach deliverance to the captives, and recovering of sight to the blind, to set at liberty them that are bruised" (Luke 4:18).

Clearly remaining poor, broken hearted, captive, blind, and bruised is NOT what God has in mind for us, so why are we willing to buy in to that? Do we really have to be so dim witted that we accept pain until it gets so bad that we finally in desperation seek Him, plead with Him, and even blame Him?

This is totally unnecessary, isn't it? Let's be honest.

When will you make time to get healed?

Beauty for Ashes

"To give them beauty for ashes, the oil of joy for mourning, the garment of praise for the spirit of heaviness; that they may be called trees of righteousness, the planting of the Lord, that He may be glorified" (Isaiah 61:3).

I am experiencing a new skin care system. It is amazing, goes deep down and repairs damage, restores a youthful skin, and makes you feel renewed! It costs money, and women buy it and faithfully apply it morning and night, because it works.

Is this vanity? No! It is maintenance; good stewardship of the body we have in this life. Do I want to look and feel beautiful? Absolutely! I want my beloved husband to rejoice in me as much as he did, even more than he did, when I was a young bride! Before the fall, Eve didn't have to be concerned with this; growing old and dying were not a part of the deal. Now, in this life, growing older and eventually going home to be with the Lord are a part of the deal. However, we don't have to do it ugly, and we don't have to do it sick!

What strikes me about the skin care system is that you have to keep it up. You must faithfully apply it every day to maintain the skin's health, or the repaired skin will not remain because the damaging elements of the environment will continue to cause problems. So women do it every day. Faithfully!

What's the point? People have no problem spending money and time consistently to restore and maintain beautiful skin, get their hair cut/colored, work out, or get a manicure or pedicure to look and feel great. The same commitment to a daily maintenance of healing can also repair and protect us from the damaging elements in this environment!

Nobody thinks you're a nut because you want your face to look good, but being healed? Refusing to give in to damaging disease? Working at it consistently day after day? Some may look at you funny when you undertake that! Tell them you have a great skin care system and they want to know all about it when they see your lovely face. You know what? If you never get sick, they may start to want to know all about that, too.

Beauty for ashes? The oil of joy? A garment of praise? That works for me. I'll stay on standing order for all of that, because I do with all my heart want to be a tree of righteousness, the planting of the Lord, that in my life He may be glorified.

Celebrating the Color of Your Eyes!

So, you trees of righteousness; you plantings of the Lord! Are you up and ready, anointed with that oil of joy? Does your garment of praise fit and flatter you? Are you easy on the eyes today?

Let's re-visit the last scripture:

"...To give them beauty for ashes, the oil of joy for mourning, the garment of praise for the spirit of heaviness; that they may be called trees of righteousness, the planting of the Lord, that He may be glorified" (Isaiah 61:3).

This scripture is a reminder to us of how it's supposed to be: beautiful, joyful, and full of praise. These are not wonderful attributes we are to strive for, they are attributes we have been given by God.

Consider this: God has chosen your eye color. He does not take it away. You may throw on some tinted contact lenses, but your real eye color remains a gift from God. He will not withdraw the gifts of beauty, joy, and praise either.

Yet some of us, and at times all of us, can be guilty of embracing the ashes, the mourning, and especially the spirit of heaviness instead. Why on earth do we do this? Because on earth we get lots of help to focus on the wrong things, that's why!

What can we do to stop it? We can KNOCK IT OFF, that's what we can do.

Rolling in the ashes, genuine, heartfelt mourning, and heaviness of heart have real appeal. They can generate attention and sympathy, and make us interesting tragic figures. They can also destroy us and the people around us. They will destroy beauty, vanquish joy, and silence praise.

Perversely appealing as they are, if we continue to cling to them we cannot be trees of righteousness, even though we were planted by the Lord, and through them He will never be glorified.

I challenge each of us to look deeply into the mirror each day, and thank God for the beautiful color of our eyes.

"Abba, thank you for choosing this lovely color for me! Thank you for dusting off the ashes, and anointing me with oil. Thank you for this beautiful garment of praise, more beautiful than anything in Nordstroms or featured in GQ. Help us to live as trees of righteousness today, and tomorrow, and all the days of our lives, never forgetting the purpose of these marvelous gifts: that YOU may be glorified!"

Inventory

Did you respond to the challenge in the previous message? Did you look into your own eyes, acknowledge and praise God for the lovely eye color He chose just for you? If you did, you may have found yourself looking deeper. This often happens when we approach God with sincere gratitude. Sometimes we are softened enough to allow new messages to enter into our spirits through the tender love we feel flowing back into us from Him.

Maybe it's time for an inventory check today. If you have been reading in sequence, you have pondered the content of over one hundred messages concerning healing.

Perhaps in the beginning the idea that God does not want us to be sick was new to you. Maybe you never knew that, and had to be convinced! As scripture and prayer presented the incontrovertible evidence, a whole new way of living was revealed to you.

The fullness of what Jesus won for us in His victory on the cross, and the role of the Holy Spirit constantly present and available to us at all times, is almost too much to take in. The facts have been there in the Word for centuries. We have read them, heard them from pulpits, and sung about them in Sunday School and gospel songs and ancient hymns. The Truth had been there all along. Suddenly it took on life and flesh. This time, the flesh was our own.

On the other hand, some readers know and have personally experienced divine healing in themselves or in others; yet the focus, some immediacy of the reality, has slipped. The world, the flesh and the devil are forces all around us crowding in to crush us and distract us. At times like that, I remember the woman with the issue of blood.

She too was pushed and crushed by the crowd, but she said, "If only I can touch the hem of His garment…" (Matthew 9:20) If we recognize what is happening to us, in the moment, we too can touch the hem of His garment, every single day.

The experiences of healing we call miracles, but they are commonplace for God. He does not want us to be ill or injured, and He will fix us when we are! Yet through His wonderful divine courtesy, God permits us to make the choice. Frustration may not be a characteristic of God, but I surely sense sadness from Him when we refuse to receive the wonderful gift He offers us, the gift that through His love cost Jesus so much.

So, how about a short inventory check today? Are you increasingly:

1) **Refusing** to accept any symptoms of pain or weakness? Do you catch it right away, with the first twinge or sneeze?
2) **Indignant** at the all too prevalent idea that it is God's will for someone to suffer for His glory?
3) **Searching** the scriptures as if you were looking for that last Hershey's kiss you just KNOW is somewhere in the messy drawer in your kitchen?
4) **Angry** when you hear of yet another person stricken with cancer, another innocent child suffering in a hospital before even having a chance to experience pain-free life?
5) **Outspoken** in your eagerness for people to know the REAL nature of God and His amazing power and love and victory?
6) **Not unduly impressed** with bad test results that don't match up with what the Word says about your health?
7) **Worry and fear free** because you have 100% released yourself spirit, soul, and body into the loving hands of the God who made you and loves you?
8) **Prompt to reject** infirmity and to seek God, the proof of scripture, and strong believers to strengthen your determination to live a healed life?

Caution: Do not be offended by this list! Consider how Jesus in the flesh, as an example for how we are to live in the flesh, was Himself refusing to accept anything less than God's will: indignant, searching, angry, outspoken, unimpressed by evil tidings, worry and fear free, and prompt to reject anything that did not match up to His Father's will.

Many, if not most, people want to live a healthy life. So often in this endeavor they spend a lot of time and attention on what to eat or refrain from eating, how and how often to exercise; keeping up with symptoms as possible indicators of health issues. Certainly these are wise precautions for us while living in the earth suits, but they clearly don't go far enough. We know more. We know a more powerful precaution and place of safety and health.

Don't we?

No Abusive Father

Throughout the centuries, animals remain true to their creation. They are born with instincts given them by God, and they continue to obey these throughout their lives. All they need has been provided. Mothers giving birth, even for the first time, know exactly what to do! Amazing! And as a friend once observed, "Any creature when it is a baby is always adorable!" How true. There is a program on TV called *Too Cute* that features baby animals. It so clear that their Heavenly Father, their Creator God, loves them and has provided for them.

Yes! Their Father and Creator is the same as ours! As the old hymn says, "...all I have needed thy hand has provided, great is thy faithfulness, Lord unto me." Animals live this. What about us?

"Look at the birds of the air; they do not sow or reap or store away in barns, and yet your heavenly Father feeds them. Are you not much more valuable than they?" (Matt. 6:26).

With the additional gifts of free will and language, our case seems more complicated than that of the animals. These are wonderful gifts, yet they can distract us from hearing the promptings of God that are instinctive to and immediately obeyed by animals. As a result of the fall, we can fail to listen or hear, and we can argue, rebel, and blame.

When we must face and experience the results of sin in the world, the sins of others as well as our own, we can blame God. We can feel that He is an abusive father, inflicting us with pain. We can cry out, not to Him but against Him, accusing Him of hideous cruelty toward His children. Yet, neither He nor the animals are hideously cruel to their children; only mankind behaves like that.

Where then is our escape? We must repent like Job in dust and ashes, acknowledging that we do not understand. We must run to Him, fling ourselves into His wonderful mercy, and rest in the safety of our loving Father's arms. He will receive us with the same tenderness we feel for the tiny kitten who trustfully purrs itself to sleep in the palm of our hand.

"But if from there you will seek (inquire for and require as necessity) the Lord your God, you will find Him if you [truly] seek Him with all your heart [and mind] and soul and life." (Deuteronomy 4:29, AMP).

We must LISTEN for the sound of His voice, because for us it is not instinct that keeps us surviving in our Father's will, but one to One communication.

"Be still, and know that I am God; I will be exalted among the nations, I will be exalted in the earth!" (Psalm 46:10).

As we walk into the love of His will, we can walk away from the abuses of mankind, and live simply and peacefully just as He created us to live.

"The steadfast love of the Lord never ceases; His mercies never come to an end; they are new every morning; great is your faithfulness. 'The Lord is my portion,' says my soul, 'Therefore I will hope in Him!'" (Lamentations 3:22-24).

Facing the "Why?"

In the face of God's eternal, bountiful, unwavering, forgiving, unlimited, matchless love for us as His children we can't help asking "why" when it comes to the sickness and disease and injury that still inflicts mankind in this life.

We do know the answer. It's in Genesis through Revelation. It's on the cross, and its solution is by the cross. We just don't want to face up to the reality that choosing evil over good affects more than the one making the choice. Since the fall, anyone who chooses to disobey the loving, power-filled guidelines and guidance of God is going to be vulnerable to these evils and make others vulnerable, too.

A person who drinks, does drugs, and then drives can cause an accident that maims or kills another person. Sexual immorality, and by that I mean God's standard, not the shifting sands of what people vote is OK because "times have changed," has inflicted hideous disease on the world. We can't deny this. One looks in grieving compassion at the children whose parents or grandparents or great grandparents made choices that resulted in AIDS, syphilis, crack babies, illegitimacy, broken homes, abortion, and unprotected innocence destroyed by abuse, physical and sexual, mental and emotional.

We must stop kidding ourselves and face reality. Is there an answer? Of course there is. The answer is in our Bibles in black and white, and especially red, and in the Holy Spirit who stands ready to help us and heal us at every turn.

We should not be surprised when we experience the "tribulation" of illness and other evils in this world. We've had fair warning that this will happen, and we've also been given the solution through protection and healing.

No other religion on earth offers both. All religions are equal? Forget that noise! They are not. They do not have the Power. Why then do we as believers so often seem to be plagued with the same issues as everyone else? If our faith has the solutions, why are we not walking in them?

Easy. It's simply because WE ARE NOT WALKING IN THEM.

Be not deceived: what we, and all of mankind sow, we shall reap. Every evil act from the modest lie to the flagrantly violent sin has an effect on us and on those around us, from generation to generation.

"Do not be deceived, God is not mocked; for whatever a man sows, that He will also reap" (Galatians 6:7).

Let's stop batting our tear-filled eyes like helpless little innocents. The world needs to see the Truth in a converted, convicted, militant Church manifesting signs and wonders so fiercely and consistently that there is no denying that there is no god like our God. Our God IS GOD. Can we be convicted of being Christians by the evidence of our lives, our health, and our determined, unflinching faith?

I love the book of Daniel, and especially the story about the Hebrew children who refused to dishonor God. They laughed at the king's decree that they worship in a different way, even when threatened with the fiery furnace. They informed him that their God laughed at fiery furnaces (Sharon's version!) and He was able to save them. Knowing that the king didn't believe this, they added "but if not," even if they burned, they would still not compromise.

"Shadrach, Meshach, and Abed-Nego answered and said to the king, 'O Nebuchadnezzar, we have no need to answer you in this matter. If that is the case, our God whom we serve is able to deliver us from the burning fiery furnace, and He will deliver us from your hand, O king. But if not, let it be known to you, O king, that we do not serve your gods, nor will we worship the gold image which you have set up'" (Daniel 3:16-18).

They survived, and so can we. God is no respecter of persons; what He does for others, He'll do for you! Are you willing to throw the "Why?" back into the Enemy's teeth? After all, the fiery furnaces are for him, not for us.

Answers that Work

Did you ever watch two little kids get into a heated argument? Each wants his or her own way, or the one toy, and cannot entertain the thought of anything other than getting what he or she wants! It begins with words, then shouts, then some pushing and if not interrupted by a responsible adult, it will lead to spitting, biting and hitting.

I have been watching the antics of Congress on the news quite a bit recently, since the outcome of their arguments can profoundly affect us all. Pretty similar to the kids, right? Why? Because when we try to please ourselves or other people we are headed for the spitting!

Most dangerous of all, as we listen to both sides of the argument, we can begin to understand both points of view. I may not agree with my opponent, but I can see how he or she thinks the way he or she does. Where can we go with that?

This is so often the dilemma people face about healing. What is true? What can you believe? What should determine your choices and actions?

Just like kids and Congress, listening to and pleasing other people will always be a dead end, and when it's your health, a dead end is not a happy place.

The book of Hosea expresses God's sorrow over the fact that people refuse to turn to Him. He stands ready to fill our every need out of His omnipotent and omniscient benevolence: "...I will have mercy on her that has not obtained mercy; and I will say to them who were not my people, Thou art my people; and they shall say Thou art my God" (Hosea 2:23).

Yet people turn from this saving grace to kicking sand in the sandbox, going their own way and disregarding God's direction. He says, "...there is no truth, nor mercy, nor knowledge of God in the land. By swearing, and lying, and killing, and stealing, and committing adultery, they break out and blood touches blood" (Hosea 4:1-2).

One of the saddest scriptures for me in all the Word is this: "My people are destroyed for lack of knowledge" (Hosea 4:6).

We have no excuse for lack of knowledge. We can read. We have the Word. We have the Lord. The Holy Spirit is constantly with us, ready to help. Yet we consult ourselves and other people having a vast variety of conflicting ideas about what we should do.

How can we possibly consider any "wisdom" that stands in opposition to that of Almighty God? It can be as if we have temporarily lost our minds, like the little kids in a fight. For them, we hope an adult will intervene, but God has given us free will, and as adults with that gift we must choose. He stands beside us, urging us, "Choose life!"

"I call heaven and earth as witnesses today against you, that I have set before you life and death, blessing and cursing; therefore choose life, that both you and your descendants may live..."(Deut. 30:19).

Little kids, big adults, and members of Congress would do well if we all stopped trying to rely on our own wisdom or that of others and instead committed to please God. He has all the answers, the only answers we can count on, the answers that work.

Heathen or Healed?

In Eden, mankind was safe and healthy and living gloriously in the presence of God. There was no evil, no sin, no illness, nothing but light and peace and joy. There was a tree, however, the Tree of the Knowledge of Good and Evil. Man was forbidden to eat the fruit from this tree, because once eaten, evil would enter the garden and the life of mankind.

We know what happened. In the moment, a fully blessed person contemplated listening to the "wisdom" of the serpent and chose it over the Wisdom of God. Immediately evil entered, and with it, death, and with death, all the things that can lead to death. Clearly sickness and disease are among them. All of this happened because mankind chose to put another "wisdom" in the place of the loving Wisdom of God.

I'm sorry that's the deal, and I'm sorrier that we are still doing it today, and I am sorriest that the results are exactly the same. Can't we fly back into the arms of God? YES! WE CAN!

I re-read the book of Joel from time to time, and I find it rich in "reality check." Have you seen any of the "reality" shows on TV? Check Joel out. Now there's reality for you, in all its gory wickedness and its glory. I know it is about particular groups of people in a particular historical context. Don't let any uber-scholarly person convince you that because of this it has no powerful message for us! Read it and weep, because you will see US in all our stupidity and in all our hope.

In the book of Joel, the people are in terrible danger of the heathen ruling over them because they themselves are behaving like heathens. The results are so awful that even nature is affected—the vineyards and the animals and the trees and the rivers. This should sound terribly familiar to us! We have allowed drunkenness and drugs (Joel 1:5), poor stewardship of the land (1:10-11), and boys to be given as harlots and girls to be sold for wine (3:3), and we have shed innocent blood (3:19). Joel 2:3 contrasts the Garden of Eden with the desolate wilderness we face when we move away from God's wisdom, love, and protection.

How can we expect to live healed if we condone heathen practices and ways of thinking? The book of Joel is filled with hope, and the powerful loving-kindness God offers us and pleads for us to embrace. There is simply no escaping the connection between sin, evil, and sickness, even though the connection can sometimes affect the innocent blood that is shed as the result of the choices of others rather than our own.

To choose God is to choose life. In both the Old and New Testaments it is so clear that God's will for "life" is wonderful beyond our wildest expectations, and certainly beyond our deserving. The choice, however, remains the same as the one in Eden.

Will we choose to be the heathen, or the healed?

Home to Healing

Did you ever come back home after a really fun trip or vacation, or a rough one, and sink into your own bed with a sense of total release and relief? Know what I mean? Nothing compares to your own pillow and your own sheets and blankets. It is just the best!

Did you ever know anyone who had to stay in a hospital for a while? Upon their return home, so often they fall into a deep, satisfying sleep. While away they feel, "Oh, if I could only be in my own bed!" and when we are finally there, the sleep is so deep and healing.

We once had a little cat named Dexter who had to have surgery. When we picked him up from the vet, He was a sorry little bundle of fur. He managed a faint meow when Moe picked him up, and he was able to manage a feeble kiss for me. However, as soon as he hit the house, he was a new cat! He ran around, leaping tall buildings in a single bound! I ran around after him saying, "Dexter! Be careful, you've just had surgery!" He still had the stitches, and I'm sure some pain, but he didn't notice them. He was HOME.

This is such a perfect picture of what we as believers experience when we walk away from our infirmities through the healing power of God. We COME HOME. We come home to our Heavenly Father, we rest in His arms, and nothing else matters. We can leave everything else behind, and rest in perfect peace.

Sometimes people can't be healed because they are afraid to come home. Don't be duped by that lie. The door is always open; it's ahead of you, filled with light. Love, healing Love, stands at that door with His arms wide open, ready to receive you in a big bear hug!

So run home! It's so glorious! Just ask Dexter!

Temple Maintenance

I was reminded of some important realities during a great conversation with another believer concerning healing. It had to do with the indwelling presence of the Holy Spirit within us, as an instructor, protector, healer and guide. What an amazing privilege we have that separates us from others in a remarkably power-filled way and fills us with longing to share the Good News with everyone!

God tells us, "...for you are the temple of the living God; as God has said, I will dwell in them, and walk in them; and I will be their God and they will be my people. Be separate from them, and do not touch unclean things, says the Lord, and I will receive you, and I will be a Father to you, and you shall be my sons and daughters, says the Lord Almighty" (II Cor.6:16-18).

What a marvelous thing, to be a temple of the Living God! We would never dream of such a thing, in trembling reverence of Him, yet He chooses to enter us. What a marvel and a glory! Stop for a minute and just think about this.

"To whom God was pleased to make known what is the riches of the glory of this mystery among the Gentiles, which is Christ in you, the hope of glory" (Col. 1:27).

Christ, the anointed God who became man in the flesh, through the indwelling of the Holy Spirit enters our flesh! Do you think He does this so we can endure sickness, fear, or poverty? Or do you think He does this so we can be filled with His healing and riches? Alleluia!

With this Living Reality walking around inside of us every day, we are separate from those who have not yet received it, and even MORE separate from the machinations of our enemy:

"Do not be unequally yoked together with unbelievers: for what fellowship does righteousness have with unrighteousness? What communion does light have with darkness? What concord does Christ have with Belial? Or what part does a believer have with an infidel? What agreement does the temple of God have with an infidel? (II Cor.: 6-14-16).

The Temple of God! That's me and that's you! We don't have to live like people who do not yet have this indwelling. We don't have to be fearful and weak and sick and poor and depressed and eat worms!

However, our temple may need maintenance. We must sweep out all doubt, fear, and thinking that does not line up with the Word and promises of God. Within ourselves we carry the joy of dwelling in the presence of God, as Adam and Eve experienced in the Garden, all day, every day, 24/7/365! Our temple cannot be like the rec room, the messy drawer, the broom closet. Our temple is sacred, holy, powerful, and filled with glory!

As we receive the recognition of His Presence there, we are so filled with light that we banish darkness wherever we go because He goes with us, and with Him we are the Light of the World.

How Is Your Immune System?

Wouldn't it be wonderful if, although hurtful things happened all around you and to you, they couldn't hurt you? Even when we try our hardest to stand immune from awful stuff, sometimes life deals it out to us anyway.

If bad things happened as the result of our own sin every time, wouldn't it be easier to handle? But when we've believed, and stood strong, and had faith like never before, sometimes the bad stuff still hurts. So we're just as bad off as the unbelievers, right?

Nope. In every situation, our case is different.

We know that sometimes we are attacked by unseen forces in the battle between Good and evil. The smaller case "e" there is intentional, Mr. Editor, leave it alone! Evil is a puny, defeated foe that does not have a chance against the POWER of GOOD. We know that, so our case is different.

When bad things appear to be happening to us, all around us, even in us, we turn ourselves over, once again, to the Living God. When we do that, no matter what happens, we know there is a reason, always, and the reason is always a good one.

We won't always know the reason, as Job confessed to God. Sometimes things are too wonderful for us to understand: "I have spoken about things I did not understand; things too wonderful for me..." (Job 42:3).

In God's hand, everything is wonderful, and one day we will understand how.

Even as a child I was fascinated by this kind of conflict, especially in the story of Joseph and his brothers. They were so jealous, and hated this beloved son of their father so much that they tried to kill Him and then they sold Him into slavery. That REALLY bothered me!

When in time of terrible famine and suffering they traveled to Egypt for food, they met the grown up Joseph. God had taken great care of him and elevated him to high places, because in spite of his suffering at the hands of his brothers and others, he remained faithful and obedient to God and God's laws.

Once all was revealed, the brothers broke down at the thought of the terrible things they had done to him, but Joseph said, "You intended to harm me, but God intended it for good to accomplish what is now being done, the saving of many lives" (Genesis 50:20, NIV).

"You intended to harm me, but God intended it all for good. He brought me to this position so I could save the lives of many people" (New Living Bible).

"As for you, you meant evil against me, but God meant it for good in order to bring about this present result, to preserve many people alive" (New American Standard).

God means everything for our good, even in this fallen world. He will use the most awful things to bring about the most marvelous miracles of love and redemption, over and over again. Men can do terrible things, and mean them for pain and evil. Evil, ungodly choices can be made that affect the innocent and cause terrible suffering, while carelessness can cause accidents and disease.

Praise God, our case is different when we place ourselves in the hands of God. Evil can't destroy us. No matter what, we trust and believe in those things too wonderful for us!

In doing that, many lives will be preserved because of our immunity. Both Joseph and Job lived to be hearty old men, extraordinary overcomers! So can we!

Who Is Wiping Your Bottom?

If we are wise, while we inhabit a physical body in this material world we must care for it as we would care for a little child. Think about it! You must feed a little baby and bathe it and wipe its bottom and protect it from harm.

So who's wiping your bottom now? I trust you are taking care of this yourself, and feeding yourself, washing yourself, protecting, etc. This is your responsibility.

As children grow up, with the development of their brains through language and experience, they are able to take over these responsibilities. We must do this, too; we must learn from the Word HOW to take care of ourselves in order to stay healthy, get healed, and live safely. Logic, however, has its limitations because it resides in a finite brain. We must grow beyond that. We must connect with God and grow in the Spirit.

I love watching generation after generation of squirrels and deer that invade our property throughout the year. I'll admit it, I DO put out veggie scraps and nuts and seeds. I feel like a mommy and a grandmother! What impresses me is how perfectly their Heavenly Father has provided for each of them. As scripture says, they toil not, neither do they spin. They do not have to find a parking space at the grocery store or worry about running out of cash at the register. They do not have doctor and dental appointments. They don't get drunk or do drugs. None of them has ever complained about a migraine.

My point is that our Heavenly Father has provided for us too, but even more. We are spirits! We just live temporarily in the body and reason with the soul, but we are spirits. Because of this wondrous reality, we can experience the indwelling of the Holy Spirit who will protect, guide, and heal us.

So, I invite you to take a moment today to run around Moe and Sharon's back yard. Grow up and beyond your concerns over physical issues. We are grownups; we must take charge, and when we have, we can turn it all over to our wonderful God who provides all things for His children, furry or not!

> "Bless the Lord, O my soul, and forget not all His benefits: Who forgiveth all thine iniquities; who healeth all thy diseases; Who redeemeth thy life from destruction; who crowneth thee with loving kindness and tender mercies; Who satisfieth thy mouth with good things; so that thy youth is renewed like the eagle's " (Psalm 103:2-5).

There's Always a Reason

When some unexpected and inexplicable event occurred, my mother always said, "Honey, there's always a reason." Clearly we didn't know what it was at the time and maybe we never found out, but there was always a reason.

Even atheists seem to agree, especially if they are scientists, "Matter is neither created nor destroyed." Even the term "random," although used out of unavoidable necessity, leaves us uneasy. Is it all REALLY so random? Some instinct tells us, "No." Even our atheist and agnostic friends accept the definition of God as "the uncaused Cause," "the uncreated Creator" for communication purposes.

A common folk wisdom is expressed in a song from the film *The Sound of Music*. "Nothing comes from nothing; nothing ever could…" OK, we get that. Then we face the fact that there is a reason behind illness, and there is an answer to "why me?" when it attacks.

Sometimes we know the reason. AIDS is spread when people make themselves vulnerable, or someone else takes advantage of their vulnerability. An alcoholic driver smashes into someone and maims him or her. Parents may walk away from their responsibility to protect their children. Sometimes we're just not paying attention at a critical moment. The recipient may well be an innocent victim, but there is always a reason.

It is especially important to recognize this in cases where individuals or a family seem to be earmarked for disaster. Some drama is always going on with them, one crisis after another; one accident, health issue, or trip to the emergency room after another. Why? Sometimes it is important to ask a question even when you don't know the answer, especially when you don't know the answer!

We need to find the answers. Guess where? If you don't know that after reading all these healing messages, then you're fired!

The Good News is that God has an answer. Psalm 91 is so powerful and so comforting and so practical. It tells us we can abide under the shadow of the Almighty! It says we need to say with our own lips that He is our safety, that we trust Him, and that He will deliver us from this disease or that attack.

God tells us that because we make Him our habitation, no evil or plague can mess with us. He will provide angels to help us. He says that when we love Him, He will deliver us, He will lift us up because we know His name! He promises us long life and salvation. The wisdom of man won't cut it, but the Wisdom of God will.

Read Psalm 91. Stuff keeps happening? Read it again. As Mom said, there's always a reason for the bad stuff. There's always a reason for the good stuff too!

Error Report

Ever get that "Error Report" on your computer screen, cell phone or some other electronic device? Doesn't it drive you nuts? When you "control/alt/delete" to get rid of the roadblock, you are asked if you'd like to report it. Usually I would skip that in order to get on with my mission, but eventually I figured out that if I keep doing that things never get fixed!

Our bodies are miraculously complex, yet they run far more efficiently in general than most, if not all, the latest technology. We generally don't notice this or pay much attention to it until something goes wrong, and the health error report kicks in. Just like technology, it really pays to report it to the "Manufacturer," who already knows what's wrong and is all too ready to back up His Warranty!

No matter what you or a loved one may be going through in the health and wellness area of your life right now, it would be a great time to stop and praise God for all the times things ran so efficiently that you didn't realize or appreciate what a marvelous body you were given.

Most of us have more sense about our cars, with the oil changes, the gas, the tune-ups, the taking it in for repairs in order to prevent a crisis. We know it takes time and money. If we have insurance or a warranty, we are right there, first in line, to demand what we're due when it comes to our wheels.

One morning a news program had a fun segment about our first cars, which started me thinking about our first bodies. You know, the ones we were born with? Oh, right! They are the same ones we still have. Pretty remarkable, as the years go by. These things were built to last! When something starts to rattle or smoke, that's a good time to send in the error report. Our Manufacturer knows exactly what we need, and He doesn't have to wait for spare parts to be delivered, or charge us an arm and a leg either.

I know I'm sounding flippant about something very serious. Sometimes, however, common spiritual sense is more readily available through a chuckle than a serious analysis. It's funny how we're just made that way.

My suggestion is that we take a moment to smile at God, and thank Him for the lifetime vehicle He so carefully created for each one of us, and appreciate all the things that have worked RIGHT, especially those we haven't noticed because we take them for granted. Then praise Him! God inhabits the praises of His people, we are told:

"You are holy, enthroned on the praises of your people Israel" (Psalm 22:3).

As He inhabits your praises, allow His glory to enter every cell of your body, sweep away every fear and doubt, and receive an infusion of His healing for you, spirit, soul, and body. Then let the praise reports begin!

Sickness? No, Thank You!

Being the child of parents and grandparents who lived through the Depression, I was taught to eat what was put before me. If I really didn't like something, I was directed to eat a small amount of it any time it was on the menu. In doing this, I eventually became reconciled to some of those dishes, and finally even came to enjoy them.

One day I encountered something that made me sick. In contrast to normal operating procedure, my parents informed me that I did not have to eat that! What a revelation! I could choose NOT TO!

In college I encountered the short story by Herman Melville entitled "Bartleby the Scrivener" about an employee who began to say, "I would prefer not to" to an increasing number of directions. As the story progresses, his calm resistance defeats everyone.

What does this have to do with sickness? Well, I once observed a dear friend from a family who has a very powerful ministry point her finger at someone who was trying to "live on the cheap" and command her to "STOP THINKING LIKE A BROKE PERSON!" What a revelation! I realized that the scripture which says "as a man thinketh in his heart, so is he" means that we have real choices about the way we live. The victory for sickness, poverty, and despair has been won for us on the cross, yet people persist in clinging to the lifestyle of helpless, defeated people. A broke mentality can cause us to just barely survive when we could be living in plenty.

See where we're going here? A sick mentality can keep us vulnerable in the same way. We have a choice, not because of our own worthiness and power, but because of God. It took me a while to insist, "I prefer not to" when illness threatened me. I had to wrap my mind around that very unfamiliar concept. It's unfamiliar because everywhere you look in our culture, you encounter the deeply held belief that sickness is a part of life…everyone must experience it…we are all vulnerable. It is not seen as good; oh no, we are encouraged to research it and get tested and treated for it, to spend money on medications, procedures, and hospital stays.

Sadly, many people "prefer not to" when it comes to taking steps that will get them healed! They prefer not to find strong believers who can show them the way; instead, they retreat into their own defeated ways and cling to others who think the same way. They prefer not to spend time in the Word, filling themselves spirit, soul, and body with the glorious truths that could set them free. In making these choices, they prefer to stay sick.

We can prefer to be healed, prosperous, joy-filled children of the Living God! We can prefer not to live life on the cheap or in a state of not feeling well. We can prefer victory or we can prefer defeat.

Which Bartleby are you?

The Secret Place

When I was a little tot, if I was awake I was running and talking, non-stop. Sometimes I could get too wound up, and as the grannies say, "That will end in tears!" My granddaddy was so good when that happened. He'd take me in his lap and let me listen to his pocket watch, then to his heart beating, and before long I would fall into a perfect, peaceful sleep.

Once during my teens I came home from a date that had upset me. Mom, who was usually the "go to person" on these occasions, was not home. Daddy came in and sat by my bed and talked with me. He explained how selfish and immature boys of that age could be. My big football-playing, military dad was so tender and loving. The world would not come to an end, I decided, and fell into perfect, peaceful sleep.

These two wonderful, tender men are now home with the Lord, but I have a husband. At the end of a troubling, stressful day he'll pull me into his arms after we have prayed and I'll rest my head next to his heart and hear it beat. Once when I was carrying our first baby, he commented, "Now I have my whole family in my arms!" Always these occasions end in perfect, peaceful sleep.

Why? With each of these fine men I have been loved, protected, and safe. Maybe you have had similar experiences. There is something about masculine tenderness that is different from the wonderful love of women. Yet even if you have not, you have a Heavenly Father whose arms will gather you in at any time, that wonderful place is called in scripture "the secret place of the most high" (Psalm 91). Man or woman, boy or girl, that place is available just for you, as available as if you were an only child! For God, you ARE that precious only child. You see, He only made one of you. You are special to Him, and He longs to hold you in safety next to His Heart.

Both of our babies, and their grandfathers, have beat us to heaven. Do I long for them? Yes. Do I mourn for them? No. I know where to find them. Like me, they are forever in the secret place, and I will always find them there.

Being Dead Is No Excuse

Most of us who come from the South know that the best food you'll ever eat is served after funerals. I don't mean the high cuisine two leaves and a grape on a plate food, I mean the rich, comforting caloric stuff that sticks to your ribs and has been a tradition in the family for generations. The reason it is so comforting is that it is prepared by people who see death as a part of life, and the end of this earthly part a time to celebrate!

The title comes from a book I love, which expresses beautifully the attitudes of believers concerning life and death and the transition between the two. It is filled with humor, common sense, and perspective. The attitude reminds me of the reactions to the announcement of a death of most of my kin.

We are often surprised, even when the deceased is quite elderly. Why? Because all of life, to the very end, is seen and valued in the perspective scripture gives us in the lives of those stalwart men and women therein. People lived till they died! They were not counting years, they were doing things. They were busy! Sarah was having a baby boy at ninety and then raising him to manhood. Old age is seen as prime time.

Once I wrapped my mind around the fact that you don't have to be sick or injured to die, these passages from scripture took on new meaning. It's amazing how much more you can pack into living when you're not concerned with dying, a lesson I've watched in the attitudes of people who were in the process of that adventure. The death part was just another spot on the road they, and we, travel from time into eternity. The prevailing wisdom, in scripture and in these wise people, seems to be just keep moving ahead!

"Oh, did you hear that old Mr. So and So died?" "No! Did he? I just saw him at the grocery store last week! Well, his son will have to finish that fence. When is the funeral? I'll take the coconut cake." Your life is celebrated with coconut cakes and their equivalent when you are born, have birthdays, graduate, get engaged and married, have babies of your own, get promotions, and die. Then what? Don't tell me there are no coconut cakes in heaven, or their heavenly equivalent. God tells me He has more than I can dream or imagine!

The fact that death is a part of our journey is no excuse for failure to live every minute to the fullest, vigorous and well. We can anticipate greater things beyond, and should be enthusiastically working toward them. I wonder what kind of frosting they use in Heaven.

The Best Route

There are lots of ways we can react to and handle the circumstances of life as human beings with free will. This includes issues of sickness and disease, injury and health, healing and victory. There is an easy way and a hard way. Jesus gives us credit for finding the easy way desirable:

"Take My yoke upon you and learn from Me, for I am gentle and humble in heart, and you will find rest unto your souls. For My yoke is easy and My burden is light." (Matthew 11:29-30)

So why do we pick the hard way so often?

Moe and I have discovered a fast route to our church, which is quite a distance from our home. This took us a while, but once we found it we cut our travel time almost in half, with fewer lights and less traffic. However, in bad weather there is another route less affected, which is preferable under those circumstances.

Before we discovered all this, we took the only route we knew. This is the situation for most of us when it comes to healing. We act on what we know. Trouble is, we don't know enough! Once we found out the easy way with the lighter burden, wow! We decided to travel that, and Jesus has been showing us more and more how to embrace the easy yoke and the light burden.

Suffering in the face of God's clearly stated and demonstrated desire to have us healed and whole can be the result of ignorance or the lack of exercising our faith. We can choose to take the path of multiple traffic lights and heavy traffic, frustration, and delay. We can also choose the way Jesus taught us.

Sometimes I forget, and find myself driving the long way again when I'm not paying attention! When this is about driving to church, I laugh at myself and settle down for a longer trip. When it is about sickness or health, however, I laugh at the devil and get right back in the Word and prayer.

Paying attention to where we are going and how we are getting there is hugely important. We know the best road map, we just need to open it up and follow it.

His Gift, Your Choice—Just Do It.

In the end, as in the beginning, it all boils down to a simple reality; a choice that will determine everything important about your life: spirit, soul, and body, in this world and the next.

How's that for starting out on a light note? Light it is, filled with light in the pain and darkness. It is the light of laughter and joy and healing, impervious to the fears and sadness and stress of a dark world. It is the ultimate, eternal truth. It is reality. It is what it is, no matter what you think about it, but what you think about it determines everything for you.

Even the atheists and agnostics are willing to concede a definition of God for the purpose of discussion. This includes the following properties: He is eternal (no beginning, no end), omnipotent (all powerful), omniscient (all knowing), omnipresent (always present) and benevolent (all good). As an avid student of philosophy, I enjoyed all the arguments about The Problem of Pain and so forth. (The Problem of Pain discusses the following questions: Why is there pain? Can't He stop it? If He can and won't, He can't be perfectly good. If He is perfectly good and can't stop it then he can't be all powerful...and so on.)

My final conclusion after searching every argument available in writing, the classroom, and lively debate is this: Shut up.

"Be still and know that I am God," He tells us in Psalm 46:10.

That is His loving way of saying "shut up" and hear me, listen to me, trust me! Turn off the clamor of your own logic, your own brilliant ideas, and enter into mine.

If you are not willing to do that, I can't help you and neither can anyone else. If you are willing to do it, you can live the rest of your days in an unimaginable power and peace and joy, eagerly looking forward to what lies ahead forever.

If you will accept the definition, ask the omnipresent God the key questions. He doesn't give out different answers to confuse us and make it harder! He tells us all the same thing. You can count on Him for the truth.

The truth? He created you out of a great love for you. He gave you free will. He sent His Son to die for you in order to 1) relieve you from the responsibility of being worthy enough of His great gift in the face of your dumb, rebellious, or evil choices and 2) show you how you can live in victory in the flesh of this material life, moving forward to the world to come. He sent you the Holy Spirit to actually be present inside of you, guiding you every step of the way if you will only welcome and listen to Him.

Being sick or well is a minor detail in the great plan God has for your life! Healing is no big deal for Him, and it could be no issue for you. You don't have to live in fear and pain and suffering, but you can if you choose to. Like sin, they can kill you. Is that really what you want? Is being independent such a great thing when you have to live like that? Yet people stubbornly choose it every day.

What if, in the face of resistance, this is all true? What if this is not just what I think? What if it's for real? There is only one way to find out. Ask Him. Go ahead. I triple dog dare you to ask Him! I have no doubt about what His answer will be!

Then turn your life over to Him, ALL of it! Even that piece you have been holding back. He knows about it anyway. Choose to receive the fullness of life He offers you as His free gift. When you do, you are in for a life of amazing miracles without limits, and you walk with your Father who loves you and will heal and shelter and protect you and tease you and laugh with you…for always!

Ask me how I know!

I just checked the Internet for the scripture about "choose life" and got a list of life insurance information. God has such a sense of humor! Here you go:

"Today I have given you the choice between life and death, between blessings and curses. Now I call on heaven and earth to witness the choice you make. Oh, that you would choose life, so that you and your descendants might live!" (Deuteronomy 30:19).

Better Than Wishes!

When Solomon became king after the death of his father David, God asks him in a dream, "What shall I give you?" (I Kings 3:5).

What would you answer if God asked you that question? Think about it. Would it be for world peace, as the parodies of beauty queens say in their fictional characterizations? Would it be for health and well-being for your beloved family? Remembering those stories about Aladdin and the magic lamp, about the tales of three wishes granted, as a child did you ponder what your three wishes would be?

Conniving little schemer that I was, I declared that I would wish for all my future wishes to come true! Now, as an adult looking back, I am SO GLAD that some of those wishes did not come true, because they would have/could have spelled disaster!

Solomon asked for wisdom. Immediately following God's granting him this request, it is put to the test (vs. 16-28). The final verse tells us that when the people heard about Solomon's judgment, they feared him (in the sense of honor and respect) because "they saw that the wisdom of God was in him" (v 28).

As we seek God's wisdom for our health and healing, far more important and powerful than release from pain is the revelation of God's power and love through us. What do people see in you or in me? If we are truly walking in His wisdom, they will see what the people saw in Solomon, that the wisdom of God is in us, and available to them as well.

Death

If you are a learned theologian, please hold your fire on this section. If you are a fearful person, you may want to read this one later. We are going to be looking, in the face, at something difficult to express in the limitations of human reason, language, and life in the flesh. However, tune into the indwelling Spirit, and hang on tight.

God created Adam and Eve to live forever. A bad free will choice resulted in death entering the human condition. Jesus took care of it. We can now live forever. So far so good?

With some spiritual growth and the help of the Spirit, we can become increasingly aware of the two worlds in which we live. Some of us are born with this awareness, but may not know what it is or what to call it. Others find themselves increasingly aware as they grow spiritually. Many discover it when they receive the baptism of the Holy Spirit and their prayer language. It is sometimes not identified because we experience it in a variety of ways.

For example, when living in Turkey, although neither my mother nor I spoke Turkish, we were frequently able to understand what was being said by Turkish people speaking their own language, and a few of them understood us even though they could not speak English. In another example, my little sister and her very young Turkish friends would chatter away to each other with perfect understanding, each in her own language! The adults would watch this and marvel. A third example, the South American archbishop visiting our church who spoke a language none of us could speak, expressed a fervent message to us, and my dear friend was suddenly able to translate it! As she did so, in English, he nodded, "Yes! Yes!" I knew her well. This was not something she had ever done before and to my knowledge has not done since; it was a gift for that moment in time.

Still with me? My beloved father suffered from Alzheimer's disease during the last years of his life, and was increasingly unable to communicate. Yet during that time he received his prayer language! We didn't know what it was, because we had never been taught about that. One day, he very boldly rebuked some evil outside the front door of my house. On many other occasions he sang very softly, praying in the spirit with perfect peace. It was a wonderful thing to sit with him during those times. If only I had known then what I know now!

When Daddy died, the loss left me longing for him deeply. Then one night in prayer, I became aware of him. Alive, well, in the eternal life he now lives. I became aware of my own earthbound flesh. Suddenly some truth about the great cloud of witnesses mentioned in scripture came alive!

"Therefore we also, since we are surrounded by so great a cloud of witnesses, let us lay aside every weight, and the sin which so easily ensnares us, and let us run with endurance the race that is set before us, looking unto Jesus, the author and finisher of our faith, who for the joy that was set before Him endured the cross, despising the shame, and has sat down at the right hand of the throne of God" (Hebrews 12:1-2).

"And Moses indeed was faithful in all his house as a servant, for a testimony of those things which would be spoken afterward, but Christ as a Son over His own house, whose house we are if we hold fast the confidence and the rejoicing of the hope firm to the end" (Hebrews 3:5-6).

Certainly we have heard teaching about these things, although perhaps not often and not much. The awareness of this glorious reality has been growing in me all my life. Now when a dear friend moves from the confinement of life in this flesh into the eternal liberty, I am filled with joy! So often they have lived a long distance from me, in another state or country for example, and when they "die" they are suddenly as close as my next breath.

I can say with all sincerity and conviction that my relationship with Daddy has grown tremendously, far greater as he has lived in the eternal world than when he was here with us. This glorious reality is what I long to express to beloved friends who mourn the loss of a dear one!

The sorrow that our enemy would have us feel, the sense of grief and defeat after a fight well fought to live, is needless distraction from the glory. As we prayerfully grown in our spiritual maturity, we can become so aware of the eternal life we are already living that the loss of this material life becomes an occasion to smile, like the smile that comes over us as we listen to a little baby struggling to say its first words.

"Lord, help us to grow increasingly aware of the eternal life in which we already live, as we draw closer to the end of our lives here on earth. We open our spirits to the reality of the life of our loved ones gone before us. We feel the love and joy that passes back and forth from one world to the next. We acknowledge with deep reverence the truth that we never lose a loved one, because all of us are forever alive in you. We anticipate with eagerness the day when we see you face-to-face, and them with you, forever! Amen and alleluia and amen!"

The Truth That Shames the Devil

My godmother taught me a health measure that is more powerful than I realized as a child. She said, "Sharon, always tell the truth and shame the devil!" We know that our enemy is the father of lies and the author of confusion, but are we aware of how his lying wiles can affect our health?

Think about all the misinformation out there about sickness and disease, health and healing. Tons! On television and in all media, in print, and on the lips of the clueless! The temptation of sin lures people into danger, and the lust for momentary pleasure blinds us to the sometimes hideous reality of the consequences. We make confused attempts to heal ourselves, trying one thing after another, filling our bodies and minds with doubtful or erroneous information, which we identify as "the cure worse than the disease."

Scripture admonishes us, "Cease, my son, to hear the instructions that cause you to err from the words of knowledge" (Proverbs 19:27).

Listening to lies can injure or kill us if we act on them. On the other hand, when we tell lies ourselves, we open the door to the father of lies. Is that what you want? Do you really want to OPEN THE DOOR to evil through a lie spoken out of your own mouth? Proverbs 19:9 flatly states, "...he that speaks lies shall perish."

Lies are spoken with the motive of getting something we desire, even if it's avoiding an argument by agreeing with the lie rather than standing for the truth. God warns us clearly in Proverbs 21: "A fortune made by a lying tongue is a fleeting vapor and a deadly snare" (vs. 6). "Food gained by fraud tastes sweet, but one ends up with a mouth full of gravel" (Proverbs 20:17).

Remember that it is truth that will set us free. The more that we align our thoughts, words, decisions, and choices with the truth, the safer we will be. Indulging in a lie can cost us dearly, though we may not see the connection between the falsehood we spoke and the evil that resulted, attacking our flesh and well-being.

The most dangerous place we can inhabit is one where we can no longer discriminate between truth and falsehood. When lies become as acceptable as truth, and are laughed off rather than feared, we are in serious peril.

Remember that although Satan was once the most beautiful of the angels, he wasn't the smartest, and he's no beauty now.

Making a List and Checking it Twice!

Ah yes, the approach of Christmas inspires good behavior in a marvelous way! How fitting that a birthday celebration, understood by the smallest child, should be most inspiring of good behavior, generosity, and self-examination!

Unlike Santa, God does not have a list of our good and bad deeds that He tallies up to see if we qualify for His gifts. He gives, not because of our worthiness, but because of His love. One of those gifts is health and healing. However, just like the gifts under the tree or in the stocking, we must be present to receive, and we must open them up. What a sad picture to imagine: a child sitting longingly in front of a pile of gifts so lovingly prepared for him, yet he will not open them because he fears that it is not permitted.

In one respect, a list for our own use might not be a bad idea. Have we put ourselves in a position to be blessed this year? Have we run right past the gifts God offers us, or run away from His generosity instead of to it?

Here is my list:

1) Have I put God first?
2) Have I done my best to learn wisdom and flee from foolishness?
3) Have I withdrawn from association with and the influence of people who are ungodly? (Ditto for movies, music, television, social, and other media)
4) Have I consciously sought out the company and conversation of wise and godly men and women?
5) Have I spoken health and wellness and refused to rehearse illness? Have I advertised Satan less and glorified God more?
6) Have I consistently refused fear and exercised faith?
7) Do I truly believe that God loves me and wants me well?
8) If so, does everyone I know see me as a living example?

Jesus was the gift that changed everything forever, and He still is! Striving to please Him, and following His wonderful example can encourage and enable us to move from the "naughty" list to the "nice"; as ready to joyfully receive and open ALL our gifts as a child on Christmas morning.

Hearing the Voice

The book of Samuel has special significance for my mother and for me. Many of the scriptures in this remarkable story have become part of the bedrock of my faith; they are filled with revelation for all of us.

Hannah, beloved barren wife of Elkanah, asks the Lord for a son. She promises that she will devote him to the Lord all the days of his life (Samuel 1:11). When the priest Eli hears her story, he assures her, **"Go in peace: the God of Israel will grant you the petition you have asked of Him"** (1:17). She has been fasting and mourning, but when she hears this she begins to eat, and her face is not sad any more. Why? Because she believes it!

When Samuel is weaned, Hannah brings him to Eli saying, **"For this child I prayed, and the Lord has given me my petition that I asked of Him: therefore also I have lent him to the Lord."** (1:28) She also speaks a word for us: **"There is none holy as the Lord: there is none beside thee: neither is there any rock like our God."** (2:2), and **"He will keep the feet of His saints, and the wicked shall be silent in darkness; for by strength shall no man prevail"** (2:9). What an affirmation that He alone is our rock, and we don't have to prevail by our own strength!

So Samuel is raised to honor and serve God, who is pleased and says, **"for them that honor me I will honor..."** However, in chapter three we are told that hearing from the Lord in those days was especially precious because there was no open vision. Samuel was taught to honor and serve the Lord, but not to hear from Him. Then he begins to hear the Lord calling him. The lovely story of how Eli prepares him for his personal encounter with God never ceases to touch my heart.

This is not just a story about infertility and fertility! As in all things, the material reflects a far greater significance in the eternal. Why was this so important to Mom and me?

As a little child I grew up in a praying household, so I copied what I heard. One day, however, I learned about Samuel and how God spoke to him, and that night in bed after "saying my prayers" I said out loud, **"Speak Lord, for thy servant heareth"** (3:9), and He did! From that moment on, I recognized the voice of my God, and prayer became a living reality.

The next morning I flew to Mom, so excited! When I told her what had happened, she wept, and then shared with me that when she first felt me move in her womb, she remembered the story of Hannah and devoted me to God.

There is so much here. We do not have to struggle to receive our healing or the other gifts of God, because the strength of man is not what prevails. The Holy God will keep us safe and well, and He will honor us as we honor Him. The most critical message for me, however, is in two verses:

"Now Samuel did not yet know the Lord..." (3:7)

"And Samuel grew, and the Lord was with him, and let none of his words fall to the ground." (3:19)

We must hear the voice of our Lord, receive it in faith, and be assured that God will indeed keep the feet of His servants always. If you have not had this experience yet, tonight when you lie in your bed, say in faith, "Speak Lord, for your servant hears" and I promise you, He will.

Healing—Signed, Sealed, Delivered

Our healing, and every other deliverance we will ever need, has been signed, sealed, and delivered. Have you been home to receive it? Only we can choose to be home, ready to open the door and receive all God has given us to overcome any obstacle in this life—door to door delivery at its finest! Are you home, but afraid to open the door? Get over yourself! Shut your enemy's whispers up, open that door, and sign for the package!

Are you crazy not to do that? Even scripture asks us that question! Paul pleads with the Hebrews, **"How shall we escape if we neglect so great a salvation, which at the first began to be spoken by the Lord, and was confirmed to us by those who heard Him, God also bearing witness both with signs and wonders, with various miracles, and gifts of the Holy Spirit, according to His own will?"** (Hebrews 2:3-4).

"He who has received His testimony has set to His seal that God is true" (John 3:33). See there? We must receive the gift and sign for it, setting our seal to the fact that God is true. John is pleading here with people who have just seen Jesus at work, and he's pleading with us too. We have seen Jesus at work in scripture and in life. Why on earth would we hesitate to sign for that?

A friend shared with me recently that her turning point came when she decided to let God be God and do His work instead of trying to do it for herself. She told me that this required both faith and patience, because she had to step aside and then to wait. Once she began to walk in this consistently, laughing at herself for making something so simple so hard for so long, she said she discovered that God was a lot better at being God than she had been! She can bear witness with her life now that **"He who trusts in his own heart is a fool: but whoever walks wisely, he shall be delivered"** (Proverbs 28:26).

We don't have to pay for the gift, it arrives pre-paid in full by Jesus on the cross: **"For you are bought with a price: therefore glorify God with your body, and in your spirit, which are God's"** (I Cor. 6:20).

There it is, on earth as it is in heaven, door to door!

Test Tube Faith

The book of Daniel is filled with wonderful insight into God's provision for His children, as well as humor and surprises. I get such a kick out of those cheeky kids marching around in the fiery furnace (Chapter 3). Of course they were filled with reverence at the power and glory of God...but I'll bet they, and the fourth Person with them, were also having a good hearty laugh!

This morning my attention was drawn to Daniel 1, which tells us about the deal Daniel makes with the servant responsible for feeding him and his friends. These were children of Judah, who did not want to eat the food of the king of Babylon. Daniel asked for a ten-day test during which they could eat their own food, being checked in health against the other children after that time. Results: they were clearly healthier than the others, wiser, more skillful in learning, and Daniel could even understand dreams and visions.

The verse that strikes me is Daniel 1:12, **"Prove thy servants, I beseech thee..."** In other words, test us to see if we are not better for eating our own food. The food here means more than the plate of beans! It means putting total trust and obedience in God above anyone else. It was not what they knew, did, or said that gave them protection in that fiery furnace. It was trust and obedience. When they were threatened with being cast into the fire because they refused to worship a pagan image, they immediately answered, **"O Nebuchadnezzar, we are not careful to answer thee in this matter. If it be so, our God whom we serve is able to deliver us from the burning fiery furnace, and He will deliver us out of thine hand, O king."** So he had them thrown in, and they passed the test.

We are tested daily, living as we do in a culture too often ungodly. People are watching us. There are many threats, many fiery furnaces. How do we measure up? Do we fall too easily for "the king's meat", the latest version of how we should live? Or are we like those boys in our trust and obedience? Do we laugh unafraid, as they did, at any wisdom contrary to the wisdom of God? When the chips are down, and we are in the test tube of faith...what are the empirical results?

Not just for our healing, but for everything, let us agree in thought, word, and decision with Daniel 1:20-21: **"Blessed be the name of God forever and ever: for wisdom and might are His: and He changes the times and the seasons: He removes kings and sets up kings: He gives wisdom to the wise and knowledge to those who know understanding: He reveals the deep and secret things: He knows what is in darkness, and the light dwells with Him."**

The New Normal!

Sometimes very dear, well-meaning people try to keep me from "getting my hopes up" about healing. They warn me that although yes sometimes healing miracles happen, "That's just not normal."

Maybe not for them, but healing became normal for me as soon as I figured out that it was God's perfect will. That was all I needed! I found some like-minded people, and we began matching expectations up to the promises of God rather than to fearful expectations of sickness and disease.

What happened?

Aches and pains went away.

A sneeze no longer turned into a cold, then flu and then pneumonia.

Things that were supposed to hurt didn't.

Thinks that "might happen" turned out great.

Tests all came back negative! No problem here!

Surgeries went fine and recovery was easy and fast.

I began to automatically expect God's best result instead of the world's fearful result. Then I started to insist on it. I had help, in the Word of God, the blood of Jesus, and the support of my stubborn friends, to say nothing of my husband who makes the Rock of Gibraltar look like a marshmallow.

Now in our own bodies, our family, our business family, and our church family, we anticipate health and healing, victory and joy. We take it for granted, with gratitude. We expect it. We insist upon it.

Does it ever not manifest? Yes. But THAT'S NOT NORMAL!

If this lines up with what you believe about God and His will for you, get excited! You're in line for a NEW NORMAL! Try it! You'd like it! Guaranteed!

Cling to Grace

The first chapter of II Timothy is so full of power and encouragement for us! If you are going through something really hard in your own life or in the life of a loved one, this is a resource that will give you all you need and beyond.

In verse five, Paul mentions the "unfeigned faith" he has found in Timothy's family, his grandmother Eunice, his mother Lois, and then in Timothy himself. God has given that gift to all of us, but Paul urges that we "stir it up." Unfeigned faith means faith that is not pretending.

Too many of us have tried to make up our own faith, which leads to figuring things out with our own limited wisdom, or based on the nonsense that is floating around out there. This is PRETEND faith! You know you're dealing with this when you struggle and struggle to believe in God's mercy and love and STILL want to give up and jump off a cliff!

For those who may struggle with suicidal thoughts or even homicidal ones, I do not mean to be flippant. I just want to highlight that we are being absurd when we get into this state. Let go of your own smarts and determination and throw yourself on the mercy of the God who made you. Trust me, He can handle that mess far better than any of us. He can and He will!

In verse seven, we affirm that "God has not given us a spirit of fear; but of power, and of love, and of a sound mind." I just LOVE that scripture, it's all I need to strengthen my backbone and make me stick out my jaw and get a big smile on my face all at once. I know I can face all evil, because "My Daddy is bigger than your daddy!" I can face it with full confidence. I'm not polite about it either. I mean business, and the powers of darkness know that it's not "feigned" too.

We have all this because (verse nine) God has "saved us and called us with a holy calling, **not according to our works, but according to His own purpose and grace,** which was given us in Christ Jesus before the world began." He didn't expect us to have the power. It's His job to be God, but He expects us to fulfill the purpose He created us to accomplish through His strength. Just think about it: before the world began, in Christ Jesus your purpose was already determined. Can we even wrap our minds around that? How utterly cool!!!

He has "...abolished death and brought life and immortality to light through the gospel..."

One of my favorite passages is in verse 12: **"...for I know whom I have believed, and am persuaded that He is able to keep that which I've committed unto Him against that day."** The reality of that glory is almost too much joy to bear.

How Do You Act?

A friend's small son once whispered to her about an adult man he saw, "Mommy, that man doesn't know how to act!" Those little guys are good observers, and she said her son was absolutely correct in his analysis.

The letter of Paul to Titus is all about people who do—or don't—know how to act. How we act is a real revelation to everyone around us. It also is a good safety measure in evaluating whether another person is honest and trustworthy.

For example, the Cretans in Titus 1:12 were a group of people who accepted lying as a normal part of public discussion. Quite a few of their philosophical descendants seem to be spouting off around here these days!

Titus is warned about people who allow fables or the "commandments of men" to turn us away from the truth. The kicker for me is verse sixteen: "They profess that they know God but in works they deny Him, being abominable, and disobedient, and unto every good work reprobate."

Now we know that we should not be cursing, stealing, getting drunk, or selling drugs to kids, but I think the ways our behavior can deny God go way beyond this obvious stuff. Anybody can "act nice," but we are called to "act powerful!" If we appear fearful, weak, doubtful, or helpless are we not guilty of professing to know God but in our works denying Him?

Jesus gave us a clear picture in the flesh of how we are to act, and we are given the unmerited favor of grace, His power to do exactly what He modeled for us. This is making me think hard. I pray that we may NEVER act in such a way that we are abominable, disobedient, or reprobate in good works while we think we're acting sweetly!

Do I know how to act? Lord, yes! Help me to live up to that every day! In Jesus' name, and in His example, Amen.

Fear Not—The Power Is For You!

My heart is very full with two scriptures today, scriptures that explain so much about the situation we find ourselves in on so many levels, both personal and national. They are II Timothy 3: 5 and 7:

"...having a form of godliness, but denying the power thereof: from such turn away," and "ever learning, and never able to come to the knowledge of the truth."

People in this state can be much more dangerous to us as believers than the clueless pagans or the frozen atheists trapped in the prisons of their own limited intellect.

Moe has often reminded me, "Just because you are in the garage does not mean you are a car." Showing up for church and being able to quote scripture is not the whole deal either.

Why is it that people can be in church, and study, study, study yet still deny the power of our faith, of God, of the Word? There are many possible reasons.

The one I'd like us to consider today is that sincerely clueless people can be teaching sincerely clueless students! We're sunk when limited human intellect is all we value in our search for the truth that works.

It is the Holy Spirit who is sent to be our teacher, as we read the scripture, and seek God. He IS GOD!!! Sometimes people fear the manifested power that God so longs to be the cornerstone of our lives here on earth, the proof positive to those who have no idea who they are even if they know whose they are.

When I first typed that last sentence, I accidentally typed "those who have **know** idea" and as I was correcting it I realized how apt it really was!

Even though Jesus told us flatly that He was departing so that the Holy Spirit could come to mentor and guide and teach us, people are afraid of Him and His power on this earth. They think we should not seek signs and wonders.

The scripture warns us not to be seeking magic shows, but the manifested power of Almighty God in our lives is no magic show! For heavens sake, don't fear it, embrace it!

Verses 14-17 conclude that the knowledge of scripture should ASSURE us. All scripture was given by inspiration from God for doctrine, reproof, and instruction, so that we may be "perfectly furnished unto all good works."

Are those good works the nice things even the heathen and atheists can do? NO! They are the good works only possible through the power of God working in us.

Signs and wonders? Bring them on! Let the world, your world, see the power that is only possible through God's grace, living in YOU.

Dictionary Definition

Because God has recently directed me to consider the meaning of His grace for us, I have been seeking references to grace throughout the scripture, and as a result have been recognizing truths I never even considered before. This should be no surprise to anyone! Still, it is exciting and tremendously encouraging in grasping what we are capable of doing and why.

Always curious about what the secular world thinks about words that have a particular meaning for believers, I checked Merriam-Webster: "Grace: an unmerited divine assistance given humans for their regeneration or sanctification; a virtue coming from God."

There are some secondary definitions too, more along the lines of being sweet and kindly and polite, but the primary definition is the one with the meat on it, and the others are more about its manifestations.

The manifestation in scripture is not about sweetness, it is about power. This realization has come crashing down on me as I've been searching the Word. To put it in Redneck, this ain't about sweetness, Jack! It's about getting the job done. If we are willing to accept God's grace, it will not be a time for writing Him thank you notes; it will be a time for admitting that we have infinite power to accomplish ANY job He has called us to do.

So much for this false humility of, "I am so unworthy, so weak, so helpless." Grace really shakes a backbone at us. Which we have by grace!

In the past few messages we've seen that the power is God's power, not our own. That's the "unmerited, divine assistance," as the dictionary defines. Understanding this changes our understanding of the word "grace" every time we encounter it. Titus 2:11, bluntly says that "...the grace of God that brings salvation has appeared to all men."

Earlier, in 1:16, Paul warns about the people who, "...profess they know God but in works they deny Him, being abominable, and disobedient, and unto every good work reprobate."

I used to think that being those bad things meant sinning, or hurting other people, or breaking the commandments. Now I see that it means way more than that; it means living in such a way that I am not taking the power of the grace of God and ACTING on it.

I understand that it is not a matter of grace versus works; it is a matter of grace giving us the power to DO THE WORKS, because without the power of God behind us, we will eventually find that our human strength, wisdom, and power is not enough. "Look, I'm only human!" is what people have said when they have either failed or given up. Instead, it should be the reason we are able to do marvelous, glorious things through the freely given, unmerited, powerful grace God has given us!

Paul shoots straight, and with both barrels in the Book of Titus, and then ends with these words: Grace be with you all.

I think I can close with the same. This is not a sweet closing, it is an in your face challenge: Grace be with you all. Now deal with it.

For My Healing Believing Friends

If you have been studying healing and exercising your faith in this area, I have something particular to say today.

I really believe what the scripture says about healing. I believe it 100%. No one else can do that believing for me; it is highly personal, between God and me. I can fool other people, and sometimes myself, but I know I can't fool Him! So in front of God and everybody I confidently say I believe 100%.

At the same time, I have had friends who have battled issues in their bodies. Jesus acknowledges part of that tribulation in this world, and immediately affirms that He has overcome.

I battle in my own flesh as well. A dear friend died recently, believing to his last breath that he would be healed.

So what do we make of all that? Nothing! NOTHING is as strong as the Word of God; nothing is more powerful than His love for us, and His clear desire for us to be healed and victorious in every single aspect of our lives.

I ask myself, how can I believe this so strongly in the face of the "evidence" of this world and plain old logic? The answer, I think, is faith. This faith is not wish or even hope. It is a gift God gives to us freely. We don't have to struggle to obtain it or to pump ourselves up to believe. It is just there, all the time. On a cold day, maybe at the beach, have you ever had the experience of walking into a patch of sunlight and suddenly felt that wonderful warmth? When you step out of it, you are cold again immediately, but when you step into it, you are so warm.

I know full well that my friend, now home with the Lord, kept himself in that warmth the whole way. Jesus was and is and forever will be the Light of the World, and as long as we are here in the world we need to remember to stay in that light, no matter what.

Ephesians 3:19-20 impresses on us God's will for us to really know the love of Christ which passes way beyond our limited knowledge, and to be filled with the fullness of God! Paul adds: **"Now unto Him who is able to do exceedingly abundantly above all that we can ask or think according to the power that is within us…"**

If you are serious about knowing how to handle and overcome EVERY tribulation life can throw at you, think on these things and ask the Power that is within you to give you the revelation to get the job done. I promise you He will.

I believe every one of those healing scriptures we've studied, I really do. I am able to do so because of the faith God has given to all of us. Through the power of another gift, unmerited GRACE, we can stand in the gift of faith all the time.

Standing in that reality, I can keep steady in believing the TRUTH through physical challenges and through question marks. When you truly know God, and stay in His light, those question marks are exclamation points all the way, in joy and victory. "These things I have spoken unto you, that in me ye might have peace. In the world ye shall have tribulation: but be of good cheer; I have overcome the world" (John 16:33).

Citations

[1] "Tis So Sweet to Trust in Jesus" written by Louisa M.R. Stead 1882 Public Domain

[2] "Jesus Loves Me" Anna Bartlett Warner 1860. Included in *Say and Seal* written by Anna Bartlett; Lippincott & Company

[3] "And Then Along Comes Mary" Tandyn Almer 1966 Valiant Records

[4] "Turn Your Eyes Upon Jesus" Helen H. Lemmel 1922 Public Domain

[5] and [6] *Chariots of Fire* Dir. Eric Liddell Twentieth Century Fox 1982 VHS

[7] "Come Thou Fount of Every Blessing" Robert Robinson 1757 from *Hymns and Psalms* Methodist Publishing House 1983

[8] "It is No Secret" Stuart Hamblin 1952

[9] *The Man Who Talks with the Flowers-The Intimate Life Story of Dr. George Washington Carver:* Glenn Clark: 9781614270669: Amazon.com: Books.

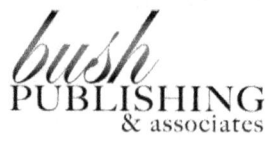

www.bushpublishing.com

www.ingramcontent.com/pod-product-compliance
Lightning Source LLC
Chambersburg PA
CBHW071603080526
44588CB00010B/1008